Frederick L. Ahearn, Jr.
Editor

Issues in Global Aging

Issues in Global Aging has been co-published simultaneously as *Social Thought*, Volume 20, Numbers 3/4 2001.

Pre-publication
REVIEWS,
COMMENTARIES,
EVALUATIONS . . .

"**F**INE SCHOLARSHIP . . . . VERY USEFUL. Ahearn has assembled a fine cohort of experts on aging who address various issues. The first section approaches them from the western industrial model perspective, but also provides an example of an Islamic traditional approach. The second section deals less with formal religiosity than with issues of spiritual transcendence in older persons. A BALANCED PORTRAIT of the aged as people rather than statistics."

Charles Guzzetta, EdD
Professor
Hunter College
City University of New York

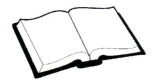

D0082200

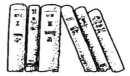

The Haworth Press, Inc.

Issues in Global Aging

Issues in Global Aging has been co-published simultaneously as *Social Thought*, Volume 20, Numbers 3/4 2001.

The *Social Thought* Monographic "Separates"

Below is a list of "separates," which in serials librarianship means a special issue simultaneously published as a special journal issue or double-issue *and* as a "separate" hardbound monograph. (This is a format which we also call a "DocuSerial.")

"Separates" are published because specialized libraries or professionals may wish to purchase a specific thematic issue by itself in a format which can be separately cataloged and shelved, as opposed to purchasing the journal on an on-going basis. Faculty members may also more easily consider a "separate" for classroom adoption.

"Separates" are carefully classified separately with the major book jobbers so that the journal tie-in can be noted on new book order slips to avoid duplicate purchasing.

You may wish to visit Haworth's Website at . . .

http://www.HaworthPress.com

. . . to search our online catalog for complete tables of contents of these separates and related publications.

You may also call 1-800-HAWORTH (outside US/Canada: 607-722-5857), or Fax 1-800-895-0582 (outside US/Canada: 607-771-0012), or e-mail at:

getinfo@haworthpressinc.com

Issues in Global Aging, edited by Frederick L. Ahearn, Jr., DSW (Vol. 20, No. 3/4, 2001). *"Fine scholarship . . . . very useful. Ahearn has assembled a fine cohort of experts on aging who address various issues. The first section approaches them from the western industrial model perspective, but also provides an example of an Islamic traditional approach. The second section deals less with formal religiosity than with issues of spiritual transcendence in older persons. A balanced portrait of the aged as people rather than statistics." (Charles Guzzetta, EdD, Professor, Hunter College, City University of New York)*

Transpersonal Perspectives on Spirituality in Social Work, edited by Edward R. Canda, PhD, and Elizabeth D. Smith, DSW (Vol. 20, No. 1/2, 2001). *"COMPREHENSIVE . . . provides theoretical and practice-oriented studies on the emerging field of transpersonal social work. The writing is both scholarly and relevant to practice. OF INTEREST TO SCHOLARS, PRACTITIONERS, AND STUDENTS ALIKE." (John R. Graham, PhD, RSW, Associate Professor, Faculty of Social Work, University of Calgary, Alberta, Canada)*

Raising Our Children Out of Poverty, edited by John J. Stretch, PhD, Maria Bartlett, PhD, William J. Hutchison, PhD, Susan A. Taylor, PhD, and Jan Wilson, MSW (Vol. 19, No. 2, 1999). *This book shows what can be done at the national and local community levels to raise children out of poverty by strengthening families, communities, and social services.*

Postmodernism, Religion and the Future of Social Work, edited by Roland G. Meinert, PhD, John T. Pardeck, PhD, and John W. Murphy, PhD (Vol. 18, No. 3, 1998). *"Critically important for social work as it attempts to effectively respond to its increasingly complex roles and demands. . . . A book worth owning and studying." (John M. Herrick, PhD, Acting Director, School of Social Work, Michigan State University, East Lansing, Michigan)*

Spirituality in Social Work: New Directions, edited by Edward R. Canda, PhD (Vol. 18, No. 2, 1998). *"Provides interesting insights and references for those who seek to develop curricula responsive to the spiritual challenges confronting our profession and the populations we serve." (Au-Deane S. Cowley, PhD, Associate Dean, Graduate School of Social Work, University of Utah, Salt Lake City)*

Issues in Global Aging

Frederick L. Ahearn, Jr.
Editor

Issues in Global Aging has been co-published simultaneously as *Social Thought*, Volume 20, Numbers 3/4 2001.

The Haworth Press, Inc.
and The Haworth Pastoral Press,
an Imprint of The Haworth Press, Inc.
New York • London • Oxford

Issues in Global Aging has been co-published simultaneously as *Social Thought*™, Volume 20, Numbers 3/4 2001.

The development, preparation, and publication of this work has been undertaken with great care. However, the publisher, employees, editors, and agents of The Haworth Press and all imprints of The Haworth Press, Inc., including The Haworth Medical Press® and Pharmaceutical Products Press®, are not responsible for any errors contained herein or for consequences that may ensue from use of materials or information contained in this work. Opinions expressed by the author(s) are not necessarily those of The Haworth Press, Inc.

Cover design by Thomas J. Mayshock Jr.

Library of Congress Cataloging-in-Publication Data

Issues in global aging / Frederick L. Ahearn, Jr., editor.
    p. cm.
    "Co-published simultaneously as Social thought, volume 20, numbers 3/4 2001."
    Includes bibliographical references and index.
    ISBN 0-7890-1439-4 (alk. paper)–ISBN 0-7890-1440-8 (pbk. : alk. paper)
    1. Aged. 2. Aging. 3. Aged–Religious life. I. Ahearn, Frederick L. II. Social thought.
HQ1061 .I88 2002
305.26–dc21
                                                           2002001476

Indexing, Abstracting & Website/Internet Coverage

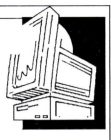

This section provides you with a list of major indexing & abstracting services. That is to say, each service began covering this periodical during the year noted in the right column. Most Websites which are listed below have indicated that they will either post, disseminate, compile, archive, cite or alert their own Website users with research-based content from this work. (This list is as current as the copyright date of this publication.)

Abstracting, Website/Indexing Coverage . . . . Year When Coverage Began

- *Applied Social Sciences Index & Abstracts (ASSIA)*
  (Online: ASSI via Data-Star) (CDRom: ASSIA Plus)
  <www.csa.com> 1998

- *BUBL Information Service, an Internet-based Information*
  Service for the UK higher education community
  <URL: http://bubl.ac.uk/> 1995

- *caredata CD: the social and community care database*
  <www.scie.org.uk> 1995

- *Catholic Periodical & Literature Index (CPLI), The* 2001

- *CINAHL (Cumulative Index to Nursing & Allied Health*
  Literature), in print, EBSCO, and SilverPlatter,
  Data-Star, and PaperChase <www.cinahl.com> 2000

- *CNPIEC Reference Guide: Chinese National Directory*
  of Foreign Periodicals 1995

- *EAP Abstracts Plus* 2000

- *Family & Society Studies Worldwide*
  <www.nisc.com> 2000

- *FINDEX <www.publist.com>* 1999

- *FRANCIS. INIST/CNRS <www.inist.fr>* 1999

(continued)

- *Guide to Social Science & Religion in Periodical Literature* **1995**
- *IBZ International Bibliography of Periodical Literature*
  <www.saur.de> **1995**
- *Orere Source, The (Pastoral Abstracts)* **1998**
- *Peace Research Abstracts Journal* **1995**
- *Sage Race Relations Abstracts* **1995**
- *Sage Urban Studies Abstracts (SUSA)* **1995**
- *Social Services Abstracts <www.csa.com>* **1995**
- *Social Work Abstracts <www.silverplatter.com/catalog/swab.htm>* **1995**
- *Sociological Abstracts (SA) <www.csa.com>* **1995**
- *Violence and Abuse Abstracts: A Review of Current Literature*
  on Interpersonal Violence (VAA) **1995**

Special Bibliographic Notes related to special journal issues (separates) and indexing/abstracting:

- indexing/abstracting services in this list will also cover material in any "separate" that is co-published simultaneously with Haworth's special thematic journal issue or DocuSerial. Indexing/abstracting usually covers material at the article/chapter level.
- monographic co-editions are intended for either non-subscribers or libraries which intend to purchase a second copy for their circulating collections.
- monographic co-editions are reported to all jobbers/wholesalers/approval plans. The source journal is listed as the "series" to assist the prevention of duplicate purchasing in the same manner utilized for books-in-series.
- to facilitate user/access services all indexing/abstracting services are encouraged to utilize the co-indexing entry note indicated at the bottom of the first page of each article/chapter/contribution.
- this is intended to assist a library user of any reference tool (whether print, electronic, online, or CD-ROM) to locate the monographic version if the library has purchased this version but not a subscription to the source journal.
- individual articles/chapters in any Haworth publication are also available through the Haworth Document Delivery Service (HDDS).

Issues in Global Aging

CONTENTS

In Memoriam   xi

PART I: GLOBAL DIMENSIONS OF AGING   1

The Future Is Aging   3
Jeanette C. Takamura

Social Security Benefits for the Family:
An Issue in Social Protection   17
Yung-Ping Chen

Retirement Patterns and Pension Policy:
An International Perspective   25
M. C. "Terry" Hokenstad
Lennarth Johansson

Who Is Responsible for the Care of the Elderly?
A Comparison of Policies in the United States,
the United Kingdom, and Israel   33
Carole Cox

Pakistan's Zakat System: A Policy Model
for Developing Countries as a Means
of Redistributing Income to the Elderly Poor   47
Grace Clark

PART II: RELIGION, SPIRITUALITY, AND AGING   77

Religiosity as a Factor Affecting Adjustment
of Minority Elderly to a Nursing Home   79
Sassy Sasson

Physical Dysfunction and Social Participation
  Among Racial/Ethnic Groups of Older Americans:
  Implications for Social Work   97
    Elizabeth M. Bertera
    Barbara Bailey-Etta

A Logotherapeutic Approach to the Quest
  for Meaningful Old Age   117
    David Guttmann

Aging, Religion, and Spirituality:
  Advancing Meaning in Later Life   129
    Gerson David

Examining Role Change: A Qualitative Study
  of Catholic Sisters Who Became Family Caregivers   141
    JoAnn Meyer Burke

Index   159

ABOUT THE EDITOR

Frederick L. Ahearn, Jr., DSW, was Dean and is now Professor at the School of Social Services of the Catholic University of America. He also holds an appointment as Tutor at the Refugee Studies Centre, Oxford University. Dr. Ahearn served on the Board of Directors of the National Council on Aging and is a member of the Global Center on Ageing founded by Dr. Daniel Thursz. Dr. Ahearn is the author of *Psychosocial Wellness of Refugees* (2000) and *Refugee Children* (1991).

In Memoriam

Daniel Thursz
1929-2000

This volume is dedicated with much affection and admiration to the memory of Dr. Daniel Thursz, a leader in the field of gerontology. Most of the authors in this volume were students, friends, and/or colleagues of his. He was also an educator and leader in the field of social work, an advocate for the poor and elderly, and an internationalist whose concerns were peace, human rights, and social justice.

Daniel Thursz, the Cardinal O'Boyle Professor of Social Work and Director of the International Center on Global Aging at the Catholic University of America, passed away January 18, 2000, a week before his 71st birthday. Born in Casablanca, Morocco, where his father was active in Zionist activities, he fled to New York with his family as a refugee at the outbreak of World War II. He received his undergraduate degree from Queens College and both his master's and doctoral degrees in social work from The Catholic University of America. During the many summers in between his studies, he spent organizing and participating in youth camp activities under Jewish auspices.

After teaching a few years at the School of Social Service at Catholic University, Dr. Thursz accepted a faculty position at the University of Maryland's School of Social Work where he soon became Dean. Under his leadership, the school grew in stature with new initiatives in community organization, social planning, clinical practice, both at the master's and doctoral levels. During this time, Dr. Thursz also became the Associate Director of Vista (Volunteers in Service to America), a program that was part of the anti-poverty strategy in the 1960s and 70s. Re-

[Haworth co-indexing entry note]: "In Memoriam." Co-published simultaneously in *Social Thought* (The Haworth Press, Inc.) Vol. 20, No. 3/4, 2001, pp. xxi-xxii; and: *Issues in Global Aging* (ed: Frederick L. Ahearn, Jr.) The Haworth Press, Inc., 2001, pp. xi-xii. Single or multiple copies of this article are available for a fee from The Haworth Document Delivery Service [1-800-342-9678, 9:00 a.m. - 5:00 p.m. (EST). E-mail address: getinfo@haworthpressinc.com].

turning to his life-long interest in Jewish service, he accepted the Vice-Presidency of B'nai B'rith International and later the Presidency of the Jewish Communal Service Association (JCSA). In both roles, he dedicated himself to peace, the care of the poor and needy, linking individuals to community so that they might have the resources and support to enrich their lives.

In 1985, Dr. Thursz took on the Presidency of the National Council on Aging (NCOA) where he advocated for policies and services to improve the lives of the nation's senior citizens. His leadership and influence were evident in the debates on social security reform, community centers, health care, and employment for seniors. When he retired from the NCOA, he returned to the School of Social Service at The Catholic University of America to begin the International Center on Global Aging that sponsored international exchanges, conferences, research, and training for professionals in the field of gerontology.

The authors represented in this volume have written their papers in memory of Daniel Thursz, recognizing his life-long contribution to social work, social justice, Jewish communal and philanthropic services, policy and services for the nation's elder citizens. This fine man, scholar, and change agent will be missed by all of us.

PART I:
GLOBAL DIMENSIONS OF AGING

Daniel Thursz, to whom this volume is dedicated, was a unique person who possessed a global vision for peace, human rights, and the needs of the aged. It was in his roles as President of the International Federation on Ageing, President of the National Council on Aging, and Director of The Catholic University's Global Center on Aging that he carried the message that all societies are enriched by their older citizens who are the repositories of values, tradition, culture, and knowledge. However, as the world's population of elders is expected to triple in the next thirty years, countries are facing crises in meeting the needs of their older citizens. Many lack the essentials of life, food, clothing, and shelter. As persons grow older, there are greater needs for health care that is not available in many cases or, if available, is so costly that older persons cannot afford it. Women, the largest cohort of elders, suffer disproportionately from poverty, isolation, poor health, and discrimination. Daniel Thursz traveled the world advocating policies that would give older persons access to work, income, health care, and shelter. Key in Dr. Thursz's vision was the empowerment of older persons as a treasure and resource for their respective societies.

The first article in this section is written by Jeanette C. Takamura, the former Director of the Administration on Aging and Assistant Secretary of Health and Human Service. In it she explores various social and moral meanings that different societies give to the rapid growth of the older population within their respective societies. These meanings influence aging policy and the type of programs that are then planned for this population. She points out that China will soon have more elders than the total U. S. population, while the number of elderly in Latin America will more than double in the next 25 years. Using the U. S. as a case example, Dr. Takamura draws the implications for aging policy and programs in the U. S.

Yung-Ping Chen, an economist and the Frank J. Manning Scholar in Gerontology at the University of Massachusetts in Boston, continues the discussion of the explosive growth of older persons in the United Sates and articulates clear policy choices for our Social Security system. He discusses the changing role of families and the effects of these changes on women and minorities in light of proposed policy changes in Social Security benefits. Two additional authors, M. C. "Terry" Hokenstad of Case Western University and Lennarth Johansson of the Swedish National Board of Health and Welfare, examine the effects of these global changes in demographics on retirement patterns and pension policy. In particular they look at how Sweden and the United States respond to the growth in older persons and the concomitant decrease in the number of workers upon the policies of work, retirement, and pensions. They discuss policy and programmatic options for dealing with this issue.

The final two papers in this section present case studies illustrating how certain countries define and handle the needs of the elderly in their respective lands. In the first instance, Carole Cox, Professor of Social Work at Fordham University, asks the question, "Who cares for the elderly?" and answers by examining and comparing the policies of Israel, the United Kingdom, and the United States. She focuses on how this responsibility is shared among individuals, families, and government. Noting that both Israel and the United Kingdom foster community care and support for family caregivers, she speculates how these approaches might shape policies in the United States. Finally, Grace Clark, the Acting Director of the International Center on Global Aging at The Catholic University of America, studies a concept from Islamic law, "Zakat," and discusses how it is interpreted and implemented in modern-day Pakistan. The zakat system is based upon the highest religious ideals in responding to the needs of the poor and elderly, especially as a means to end beggary and redistribute income. However, while Pakistan's program has demonstrated some success, it has suffered limitations due to favoritism, corruption, and governmental greed.

The dramatic demographic increases of the elderly is a global issue that raises the question of how to care for the needs of this population. Policy and programmatic approaches with respect to work, retirement, pensions, health care, and family responsibility have been debated most everywhere in the world. These articles clearly portray global examples of the key dimensions of aging in developed and underdeveloped countries throughout the world.

The Future Is Aging

Jeanette C. Takamura

SUMMARY. The social and moral meanings of aging and of being an older person are evolving within an increasingly global context. Although there are differences that can be drawn between developed and developing nations, these meanings appear to be differentiated by variables such as gender, race and ethnicity, living arrangements, and age cohort. However, the legitimacy or dominance accorded some of the meanings will likely be dependent upon the ideological beliefs of those who are deemed experts or who wield influence in policy circles. Meanwhile, the resolution of many of the most pressing aging policy issues will be compelled by the sheer demographics of aging and confounded by the extent to which ideological perspectives are intractable. *[Article copies available for a fee from The Haworth Document Delivery Service: 1-800-HAWORTH. E-mail address: <getinfo@haworthpressinc.com> Website: <http://www.HaworthPress.com> © 2001 by The Haworth Press, Inc. All rights reserved.]*

KEYWORDS. Aging, longevity, social and moral meanings

In diverse cultures and during different eras, aging and being an older person have held varying social meanings. Today, ours is a global soci-

Jeanette C. Takamura, PhD, is Assistant Secretary for Aging, 1997-2001, U.S. Department of Health and Human Services, c/o 403 Mamaki Street, Honolulu, HI 96821.

The ideas expressed herein do not represent the views of the U.S. Department of Health and Human Services or of the Administration on Aging. They are solely those of the author in her personal capacity.

[Haworth co-indexing entry note]: "The Future Is Aging." Takamura, Jeanette C. Co-published simultaneously in *Social Thought* (The Haworth Press, Inc.) Vol. 20, No. 3/4, 2001, pp. 3-16; and: *Issues in Global Aging* (ed: Frederick L. Ahearn, Jr.) The Haworth Press, Inc., 2001. pp. 3-16. Single or multiple copies of this article are available for a fee from The Haworth Document Delivery Service [1-800-HAWORTH, 9:00 a.m. - 5:00 p.m. (EST). E-mail address: getinfo@haworthpressinc.com].

ety with more shared realities generated in real time by telecommunications networks and by multinational corporations whose employees design, build, and market products that are well-known in marketplaces around the world. Another social reality that is a growing global phenomenon is population aging and longevity. However, unlike Generation Xers and others who might be viewed as members of a technologically proficient subculture with a common base of technical knowledge and a complex language, older persons in developed and developing nations may have advanced age in common, but may otherwise be characterized by tremendous diversity.

The extent to which the life situations of older persons around the world and thus the meanings of aging and of being an older person differ in a global context is easily illustrated. In AIDS-torn Africa, where many elders have no alternative but to parent their grandchildren, aging does not mean retirement or a less demanding life. In Asia, where urbanization and modernization are attracting young people to urban centers, traditional expressions of deep-rooted Confucian values of filial piety are being severely challenged. In Latin America and much of the developing world, the role of older persons may seem to be in limbo as nations attempt to transition to full economic and social development, giving emphasis to the health and welfare of infants and children.

The discussion of the range of everyday needs that must be addressed by government policies and programs were articulated in stark terms at the September 1999 Fourth Global Conference of the International Federation on Ageing. Some ministers of aging agencies and bureaus in developed nations with growing numbers of older persons expressed concern about how to ensure that economic security, health, and long term care infrastructures and systems are responsive in their aging societies. Other ministers from developing nations spoke about the need to develop programs that can address basic life and survival needs. A minister from an African nation described her country's efforts to urge families to set aside some of their own food supply–"one banana"–for collection and redistribution to poor elders. She also expressed interest in the congregate meals programs in the United States. Through Title IIIC-1, Congregate Nutrition Services, and Title IIIC-2, Home-Delivered Nutrition Services, of the Older Americans Act, millions of at-risk older persons in the United States are provided with congregate and home-delivered meals, in most cases five days a week. However, even with such programs in place, funding constraints have resulted in an inability to support the receipt of meals by many older persons.

This article examines the evolving meanings of aging in light of the growth of the older adult population, the frequently competing values that are reflected in these emergent meanings, and their implications for aging policy and program perspectives and initiatives. The latter is related narrowly to the discussion of policy options from a U.S. perspective. It is essential to note, however, that aging issues in this country will be shaped inevitably by global aging because of the sheer number of older persons that may be expected worldwide. China alone will have more old persons in the near future than the total U.S. population. In Latin America and the Caribbean, the number of persons 60 years of age and older will increase from 42 million to more than 97 million over a 25 year period (Takamura and Justice, 1999).

WHAT IS "OLD" AND WHAT DOES IT MEAN TO BE AN OLDER PERSON?

Within the American context, aging and being an older person have been regarded historically with ambivalence. Achenbaum examined some of the social meanings of aging and of being an older person that have been dominant since the founding years of the nation, applying these to analyze societal aging. Noting that in the early American centuries individual aging was often equated with maturation and that being older was commonly related to wisdom, he also observed that new fascination with the vigor and vitality of youth accompanied the period of societal redefinition which ushered in the 20th century. He argues that the preoccupation with youth that emerged may have contributed to the growing tendency to use negative images of older persons. No longer seen as sages, older persons began to be characterized as ". . . fuddy-duddy, geezer, sissy, stuffed shirt, cold feet . . . ," devalued and disrespected as irrelevant, odd, impotent, or as past their prime. Longevity, on the other hand, appears to have borne more positive meanings, with early references to the individual achievements and dignity of centenarians and to their being testament to the existence of a moral political order (Achenbaum, 1986).

In the decades just preceding the start of the 20th century, the age of 65 was introduced by Chancellor Otto von Bismarck to demarcate "old age" in Germany's first pension plan. The United States followed suit decades later in 1935, when the Social Security Act was enacted into law with age 65 as the eligibility age for the program.

Because of the extension of longevity and the anticipation that the number of centenarians[1] will increase significantly, there have been those who have argued that the age of eligibility for Social Security, often used as a proxy for old age, should be raised. Some have suggested that it should be raised progressively from 65 currently to 76.4 years of age in 2050 to keep pace with the extension of the human life span in the years ahead (Peterson, 1999). Underlying this perspective is a sense that the continued dependency of growing numbers of older persons upon the Social Security program is neither fiscally sustainable nor morally defensible and that they are an economic burden. Arguments to the contrary have ranged from noting that modifications in the eligibility age would be unjust, penalizing individuals employed in jobs that are physically demanding and placing them at greater risk of disability, to references to the substantial contributions made over lifetimes by older persons (Kalache, 1999). Though it does not address the age of eligibility issue directly, a 2000 amendment to the Social Security Act was enacted and raised the earnings limit of persons 65 to 69 years of age, enabling individuals in this age range to be employed without the benefit penalties that previously existed.

Rowe and Kahn noted recently that many of the most resilient myths in recent times about aging and older persons can be captured in the following assertions (Rowe and Kahn, 1998):

Myth #1: To be old is to be sick.
Myth #2: You can't teach an old dog new tricks.
Myth #3: The horse is out of the barn.
Myth #4: The secret to successful aging is to choose your parents wisely.
Myth #5: The lights may be on, but the voltage is low.
Myth #6: The elderly don't pull their own weight.

Each assertion presents a simplistic, distorted view of aging and of being an older adult. For example, while older adults are more likely to have chronic illnesses than are young persons, many of which are preventable or can be successfully managed, the rate of disability among older persons has been declining for a number of years (Manton et al., 1993). Approximately 83% of older Americans do not have functional limitations. Only five percent of all older Americans are nursing home residents at any one time. Twelve percent have functional limitations, but reside in the community (Komisar, Lambrew, and Feder, 1996). The vast majority of older persons are independent, reside in the community, and assess their own health as being relatively good (National Council on Aging, 2000).

In a speech delivered at the United Nations, Hagestad averred that there are "too many 'd-words' in conversations about aging, at least in English. . . . Decline, dementia, dependency, disease, disability, . . . disaster and deluge" (Hagestad, 1999). This may be a valid observation given the extent to which Medicare and Social Security reform, concerns about Alzheimer's Disease, long term care, and family caregiving have dominated national policy discussions and research related to older persons. Because these are critical issues that engender tremendous fear and anxiety among older Americans and their families, and significantly impact upon their quality of life, such a preoccupation may be both essential and constructive in some regards. To the extent that it generates more interest in younger and older generations in healthy lifestyles that promote health and help to prevent disease, it may contribute in the long run to better individual and community awareness and thus improved health outcomes. To the extent that such focus distracts and blocks out the spectrum of meanings related to aging and to being an older person, Hagestad is correct. It diminishes older individuals and disallows the consideration of evidence that growing numbers of older persons are aging successfully and are actively, vitally engaged in community and family life.

Although there is no doubt that ageist perspectives persist, a 2000 national survey of more than 3,048 adults of all ages in the United States has presented new evidence of possibly widely held perspectives of aging, old age, and of being an older American. The study discovered that 41% of those surveyed see decline in physical ability–not a set number of years–as the marker for the beginning of old age. Thirty-two percent saw the decline in mental functioning and 14% regard a specific age as the key marker for defining "old age." Related to this, one-third of older American respondents 70 years of age and older see themselves as middle-aged, as did 45% of those interviewed between 65 to 69 years of age. When compared with results from a similar survey conducted in 1974, it appears that older persons are less likely to be seen as "very warm and friendly" or as "very open minded and adaptable" than nearly a quarter of a century ago. However, the more than a century old characterization of older persons as "geezers" appears to be on the wane. Reflecting either a beneficent attitude or an understanding of the declining economic security of persons over a long life span, ninety-two percent of all survey participants of all ages took issue with the statement that "old people are greedy geezers." Eighty percent of the respondents concurred that "older people get too little respect from younger people" (NCOA, 2000). The results of the survey may suggest that the existence of an intergenerational schism is at best mythical. They may also suggest that in terms of moral identity older persons are less likely to be viewed in negative terms. Finally, they may illustrate that there is growing truth to the 1999 United Nations International Year of the Older Person pronouncement that we are on the verge of entering "a new age for old age" (Alvarez, 1999).

If we are indeed entering a new age for old age, then it is important to not color the older adult population, globally or here in America, in homogeneous tones. While many older Americans are faring better than previous generations of elders, aging and being an older adult are clearly experienced differently by several segments of the older adult population. Respect, self-determination, autonomy, or independence may be less evident for older women and for minority elders, who tend more likely to be poor, undeserved, and to suffer health disparities.

It is in the examination of data about the life situation of older women that the need to engage in subgroup analysis becomes most apparent. Strictly in terms of numbers, older women outnumber older men. From age 65-69, the sex ratio of older women to older men is 118 to 100. At age 85+, there are 241 women for every 100 men (AARP and the Administration on Aging, 1999). Aging is indisputably a women's issue, and it appears that generalized meanings of aging do not hold true for women as a subpopulation.

It is also through the examination of data that moral judgments and values purportedly held by society about aging and being an older person can be best scrutinized for their generalizability. For although fewer older persons (11%) are below the poverty line, the quality of life of older Americans clearly is differentiated by gender, race and ethnicity, marital status, and by such life circumstances as living arrangements. In terms of poverty alone, marital status, being a widow or divorced, living arrangements, increased age, and race have consistently proven to be strong determinants of poverty (Browne, 1998). For example, older women tend to be poor more often (12.8%) than older men (7.2%), with African American women who live alone experiencing the highest poverty rates (49.3%) (AARP and the Administration on Aging, 1999).

Unfortunately, increased risk during the later years of life is the result of well-known gender-based inequities with which younger and older women in the workforce and women who are homemakers must contend. Decent salaries and wages while employed, pensions, and other retirement benefits are prerequisites for economic security, but also for access to health care and social participation and engagement. Over the long term, the bearing of significant caregiving responsibilities–generally by women–for older family members may emerge as another good predictor of poverty and of health risks in the later years.

The extent to which the meanings of aging and of being an older person in the United States are colored by ethnicity and race will grow in the decades ahead. By 2050, 36% of all elderly persons in the United States will be from a minority racial or ethnic group (Federal Interagency Forum on Aging Related Statistics, 2000). Like the general female population, there are more elderly women of color than there are elderly men of color and more of them are widowed than their male counterparts. At the heart of some of the stresses experienced by elderly minority women may be the clashing of traditional and emergent roles. The new role of an elder in the context of their acculturating family and the community may be much different and lacking in the respect and reverence inherent in more traditional roles. This appears to be the case among elderly Asian American women, for example, who have markedly high suicide rates, that some attribute to a loss in old age of a valued position and role within their families and their ethnic communities (Pascual, 2000). The emotional terrain that must be traveled by minority elderly women between feeling respected and feeling isolated and unsure of one's place cannot be underestimated.

Larger in number than any preceding generational cohort, the baby boom generation is expected to redefine aging and what it means to be an older adult. Roszak is particularly optimistic, arguing that the boomers will play a significant role in strengthening our social capital through contributions of their vitality and talent in their older years (Roszak, 1998). Predicting the values that might be attached to aging by baby boomers is no easy task, however. The 76 million individuals who are included in this generation were born between 1946 and 1964, a relatively long expanse of time during which the nation and the world were undergoing rapid, multidimensional changes. Thus, the within-generation differences may be as noteworthy as how boomers differ from the generations before and after them. In this regard, they are not unlike those who make up the elderly population today. They are an extraordinarily diverse group who have demonstrated the ability to raise questions about the most basic of social institutions–the family, giving it some variant meanings that, though not formally legitimized, are gaining some conventional acceptance.

One of the questions for the future will be the role and impact of spiritual and religious activities in relation to the elderly population in

America. A growing number of researchers have explored the effects of religiosity and church attendance among older adults. In general, there appears to be good evidence of a positive relationship between church attendance and religiosity by older persons and their psychological well-being and health status (McFadden, 1995; Levin and Chatters, 1998). Similarly, several studies have evidenced a positive relationship between the variables religiosity and church attendance on life satisfaction (Cox and Hammonds, 1988; Morris, 1991). Other studies have found similar beneficial effects among African American elders (Walls and Zarit, 1991; Krause, 1992).

Clearly, there will be a number of forces that will help to construct social meanings of aging and of being an older person that are likely to be multidimensional. Whether one sees the baby boomers as bringing forward a new day of altruism and community or as being the cause of fiscal crises and societal disequilibrium, the legitimacy accorded some of these meanings will inevitably reflect and stem from the ideological, philosophical beliefs of those interacting with issues that affect older persons. It is possible that the dynamics and development of societal processes and population diversity in the future will result in a series of structural and other adjustments over time as numerous perspectives and interests are mediated. For those who are gerontologists and who are concerned as well about the families of older persons, participation in the construction of social realities about aging will be important. It will be important in order to prevent the dominance of moral meanings that could result in the devaluation of the first large elderly population the world has ever seen.

POLICY ISSUES FOR THE 21ST CENTURY

Many of the most pressing aging policy issues facing decision makers in the United States are surrounded by a sense of urgency because of existing or anticipated strains upon public and private sector programs and service delivery systems. This sense of urgency has also been heightened by the projected costs associated with the coming of age of 76 million members of the baby boom generation. Because this will begin to occur in 2011, it is likely that all of the major issues related to the aging of America will top the domestic policy agenda throughout the current decade and beyond.

Dire peril has been forecast by some, if specific public policy changes are not made and if the roles of government, the private sector, and the individual and family in relation to older adults are not altered in the near future (Peterson, 1999). But Estes has asserted that any sense of crisis is socially constructed and that how issues and solutions are cast and perceived are very much shaped by the value orientations of those who have gained legitimacy as "experts" or are in decision-making positions (Estes, 1979). Options selected from the marketplace of perceived societal alternatives are inescapably value laden. What then are the moral principles that will guide the choices that must be made? With the exception of the aspirations for the quality of life of all older Americans set forth in Title I of the Older Americans Act, there are few specifically articulated.

A divergence of ideology and philosophy have clearly reflected at least two schools of thought in the Social Security and Medicare reform debates that have been occurring over a number of years. One perspective holds that the Social Security program must be modernized and that the continuation as-is of one of the United States' largest public programs thwarts the potential of older Americans to earn the highest possible retirement income benefits through a private investment approach. The argument by these proponents has pointed to the retirement income earnings possible if funds were to be invested in the private market, presuming that the individual is schooled in the art and science of investing. Moreover, they hold that individual choice and self-determination are better honored and enabled by privatization. Those who disagree are not as sanguine about the potential of the market to provide retirees with adequate, reliable financial resources. They have argued instead that market volatility could create social insecurity among many older Americans who are most in need of a protected, reliable retirement income–i.e., women, minorities, and persons who were in lower paying jobs during their work years. They have also referred to generally unrefuted evidence that the reliability of the Social Security program has kept many older women from falling below the poverty line.

As noted earlier, the lengthening of the life span of the U.S. population has also led to some reform advocates to call for the raising of the age of eligibility for Social Security. In addition to the considerations noted at the beginning of the article, other issues that have been raised in relation to the need to modernize Social Security have included the dramatic shift in the worker to retiree ratio that has occurred over several decades. Presumably, eligibility at an older age might ensure that the huge store of human capital that older workers represent would not be lost from the work place. That is, an older age of eligibility might provide a stronger incentive for workers to remain in the work force for more years, as might employers' interests in retaining persons with the right skills, irrespective of age. Ironically, this interest exists concomitantly with trends in recent times to downsize organizations and to entice higher salaried older employees to retire. It also exists within an emergent reality in which early retirements are not unusual among even younger adults, particularly those who have reaped the riches of the high tech industries. And, although he recognizes that there are numerous variables that could affect the work force participation of older persons, Friedland points to the fact that formal policies have encouraged continued work by older individuals but that employers continue to perceive greater advantages in employing younger workers (Friedland, 2000).

Far more complex than the Social Security reform debates are those which revolve around the modernization of the Medicare program and around the growing and costly long term care needs of an aging population. The need to assist a significant number of older Americans with the cost of prescription drugs is an undisputed item of high priority on the nation's policy agenda. There is no consensus, however, around the specific target population and the structure or expansiveness of the benefits and around the delivery system through which the benefits should be received. Here again, ideological perspectives weigh in heavily, with divergent beliefs about the role and the responsibility of the individual, of government, and of the private sector.

The discussions about the long-term care needs of an aging population are complex and multifaceted. There is consensus about the cost of long term care being too exorbitant to be shouldered by most elderly Americans and their families. There is consensus about the need for an increased supply of home and community-based long-term care services. There are concerns about lack of integration of the acute and long term care systems and about the quality of care received by those who are unable to care for themselves. Increasingly, there is concern about the adequacy and the stability of the labor force. However, there has not been resounding agreement over any comprehensive strategy to help individuals and families cover these costs, whether care is provided in the home, community, or in institutions. As in the case of the early efforts of the Clinton Administration to reform health care, ideological perspectives are in apparent conflict. There is accordingly a departure of opinions among numerous constituencies on the roles and responsibilities of government, the private sector, and the individual and on the specific financing mechanisms and delivery systems.

Much of the activity and the progress in long-term care have occurred at the state and local level particularly through the use of Medicaid waivers. However, the Clinton Administration, in support of family caregivers of older and younger persons with functional limitations, proposed several significant federal initiatives in 1999 and 2000. These proposals reinforce a growing awareness of the important roles played and the contributions made by family members in support of relatives who are unable to care for themselves. They have been presented as offering initial steps in the work to establish a more comprehensive and integrated national policy related to long term care. While modest, they offer much needed support for and a beginning acknowledgment and a formal legitimization of the dominant role of the family in the provision of long term care. If the proposals are enacted and followed in the near future with supportive health and labor policies, they will affirm the value of the efforts of family caregivers–most of whom are women–who are saving the nation billions of long term care dollars. Without these, gender-based inequities will continue and potentially be exacerbated. With supportive policies, women will have a chance at financial security and optimal health in their own advanced years.

One of the other proposals in the package of long term care proposals calls for dispelling the myth that Medicare provides long term care protection. Some older and younger Americans have falsely believed that Medicare provides long-term care benefits. This may be due in part to the relatively liberal use of Medicare home health benefits by care providers prior to the tightening of program regulations in the late 1990's to ensure the provision of home health care for short-term recuperative and rehabilitative health care. It was also due to the lack of any other reliable, widely available financing mechanism that could be utilized by health care providers and families to meet the need for and the costs of home health care.

Three proposals related to assistance with the cost of long term care. One administration proposal called for a tax credit initially of $1000, later revised to $3000, for a family caregiver or the individual receiving long term care assistance from a relative. Tied to income levels, this initiative was offered to provide a measure of financial support to the caregiver or the care recipient living at home or in the community. A second proposal, which was enacted into law as the Long Term Care Security Act in 2000, establishes a pilot program in the federal government offering unsubsidized private long term care insurance options to federal employees and their families. A third proposal, proposed by Congress and also enacted into law, provides tax credits to all taxpayers that purchase private long-term care insurance. Each of these offers some segments of the American population with a degree of protection. They provide choice and enable citizens to take individual responsibility for potential risks. However, there are concerns that have been expressed about the majority of the population that, for example, might be unable to afford the premiums or who might have pre-existing health conditions that disqualify them from being good risks for private sector options. Issues have also been raised by regulators and consumers about marketing practices (Stone, 2000). Those who wish to provide security to the largest possible number of individuals and families thus remain concerned. Whether this will mean that a true public-private sector alternative can gain ground in the future is yet to be determined.

The Clinton Administration also proposed to establish the National Family Caregiver Support Program, which will establish a system of support for family caregivers. Deliberations and final negotiations on the reauthorization of the Older Americans Act (P.L. 106-501), through which the program is authorized, were concluded during the final hours of the Second Session of the 106th Session. As offered by the Administration on Aging in the Department of Health and Human Services, the national program will provide a beginning number of approximately 250,000 family caregivers of older persons and grandparent caregivers of grandchildren with supportive services which they identified as necessary. These include information, assistance in getting to support services, caregiver education, caregiver support groups, counseling, respite, and other support to help sustain the individual providing care. The nationwide Aging Network of state and local agencies on aging will design and manage the program to meet the needs of families within their jurisdictions.

CONCLUSION

There will be no lack of issues to address as America prepares for the graying of its population. The debate around the role of government versus individual and family responsibility, about equity, parity, self-determination and autonomy, choice, respect and dignity, access, responsiveness, quality, efficiency, affordability, security, and other issues will heighten in the years ahead. This is inevitable as efforts continue to modernize Social Security, reform Medicare, and design and build health and long term care financing and service systems that can meet emergent needs. This is also inevitable as combined forces of the public health agencies and institutions pursue the elimination of health disparities in ethnic minority groups by the end of the first decade of this new century. Focused attention and committed action in this area would mean that minority Americans would not continue to be marginalized and neglected by systems of care.

The mental health needs of Americans of all ages also may be expected to rise on the public policy agenda. With this, must come focused attention to the incidence and prevalence of depression among older Americans and to the high rates of suicide among specific groups of elderly persons such as older white men and older Asian American women. Concomitantly, breakthroughs in science and technology will simply multiply the bioethics issues that must be considered. The moral implications of organ transplantation, possible interventions in genetically linked diseases, issues of confidentiality, access to benefits by persons at genetic-risk are just a few of the concerns that have already arisen. In almost every case, future policy makers will be called upon to reconcile fiscal constraints with legal mandates, a stronger base of empirical evidence, and the competing interests and expectations of numerous, oftentimes single-issue constituencies and to determine how these queue in the national interest.

One thing is clear. In terms of the public policy agenda, the impact of population aging and longevity will be significant. The future is, in many regards, aging.

NOTE

1. According to the U.S. Census Bureau, from 65,000 centenarians in 2000, the number of persons 100 years of age and older will grow to 381,000 persons in 2030. See U.S. Census Bureau, accessed online at <www.census.gov/population/www/projections/natproj.htm>.

REFERENCES

AARP and the Administration on Aging, U.S. Department of Health and Human Services. (1999). *A profile of older Americans: 1999*. Washington, DC: AARP.

Achenbaum, W.A. (1986). America as an aging society: Myths and images. *Daedalus, 115* (1):13-30.

Alvarez, J. (1999). Comments made during the United Nations International Year of the Older Person.

Browne, C.V. (1998). *Women, feminism, and aging*. New York: Springer Publishing.

Cox, H. and A. Hammonds. (1988). Religiosity, aging, and life satisfaction. *Journal of Religion and Aging, 5* (1-2):1-21.

Estes, C. (1979). *The aging enterprise.* San Francisco: Jossey-Bass Publishers.

Federal Interagency Forum on Aging Related Statistics. (2000). *Older Americans: Key indicators of well-being.* Washington, DC: U.S. Government Printing Office.

Friedland, R. (2000). *Will baby boomers work more years than their parents did?* Washington, DC: National Academy on an Aging Society.

Hagestad, G. (1999, October). *Towards a society for all ages: New thinking, new language, new conversations.* Paper presented at the United Nations, New York.

Kalache, A. (1999). Active aging makes the difference. *Bulletin of the World Health Organization, 77* (4):299.

Komisar, H.L., J.M. Lambrew, and J. Feder. (1996). *Long term care for the elderly.* New York: The Commonwealth Fund.

Krause, N. (1992). Stress, religiosity, and psychological well-being among older blacks. *Journal of Aging and Health, 4* (3):412-439.

Lewin, J.S. and L.M. Chatters. (1998). Religion, health, and psychological well-being in older Americans. *Journal of Aging and Health, 10* (4):504-513.

Manton, K.G. et al. (1993). Estimates of changes in chronic disability and institutionalization, incidence and prevalence rates in the United States elderly population from the 1992, 1984, and 1989 National Long Term Care Surveys. *Journal of Gerontology, 48*:S153.

McFadden, S.H. (1995). Religion and well-being in aging persons in an aging society. *Journal of Social Issues, 51* (2):161-175.

Morris, D.C. (1991). Church attendance, religious activities, and the life satisfaction of older Americans in Middletown, U.S.A. *Journal of Religion and Gerontology, 8* (1):81-86.

National Council on the Aging. (2000). *Myths and realities of aging 2000.* Washington, DC: National Council on the Aging.

Pascual, C. (September 14, 2000). Why more elderly Asian women kill themselves. *Washington Times,* D1, 6.

Peterson, P. (1999). *Gray dawn: How the coming age wave will transform America–and the world.* New York: Times Books.

Rosznak, T. (1998). *America the wise: The longevity revolution and the true wealth of nations.* New York: Houghton Mifflin.

Rowe, J.W. and R.L. Kahn. (1998). *Successful aging.* New York: Pantheon Books.

Stone, R.I. (2000). *Long-term care for the elderly with disabilities: Current policy, emerging trends, and implications for the twenty-first century.* New York: Milbank Memorial Foundation.

Takamura, J.C. and D. Justice (1999). Creating promises out of longer life: The Americas in the 21st century. *Perspectives Health: Journal of the Pan American Health Organization, 3*:2:2.

Walls, C.T. and S.H. Zarit. (1991). Informal support from black churches and the well-being of elderly blacks. *The Gerontologist, 31* (4):490-495.

Social Security Benefits for the Family:
An Issue in Social Protection

Yung-Ping Chen

SUMMARY. Demographic changes in society have clear implications for the U. S. Social Security system. Changing familial relationships will affect the scope and value of Social Security protection that will require policy changes as well. In reporting the changes in family structure, this analysis also discusses implications for Social Security benefits and the effects on minorities and women, and calls attention to policy proposals. *[Article copies available for a fee from The Haworth Document Delivery Service: 1-800-HAWORTH. E-mail address: <getinfo@haworthpressinc.com> Website: <http://www.HaworthPress.com> © 2001 by The Haworth Press, Inc. All rights reserved.]*

KEYWORDS. Social Security, elderly women, social policy, family structure, demographic changes

The effect of demographic change, in the form of population aging, on the Social Security program is widely discussed. But the effect of another demographic development, that of changing family structure, on

---

Yung-Ping Chen is the Frank J. Manning Eminent Scholar in Gerontology at the University of Massachusetts, 100 Morrissey Avenue, Boston, MA 02125-3393.

This paper is based on a presentation given at the annual Congress of International Institute of Public Finance in Moscow, August 26, 1999, and notes of presentations at The Urban Institute in Washington, DC, September 23, 1999 and June 19, 2000.

[Haworth co-indexing entry note]: "Social Security Benefits for the Family: An Issue in Social Protection." Chen, Yung-Ping. Co-published simultaneously in *Social Thought* (The Haworth Press, Inc.) Vol. 20, No. 3/4, 2001, pp. 17-23; and: *Issues in Global Aging* (ed: Frederick L. Ahearn, Jr.) The Haworth Press, Inc., 2001, pp. 17-23. Single or multiple copies of this article are available for a fee from The Haworth Document Delivery Service [1-800-HAWORTH, 9:00 a.m. - 5:00 p.m. (EST). E-mail address: getinfo@haworthpressinc.com].

Social Security has not been generally recognized. Because the program not only provides income to retired and disabled workers but also to their eligible dependents and survivors (auxiliary beneficiaries), changing familial relationships will affect the scope and value of Social Security protection. If Social Security's benefit provisions for the family are unchanged, then the program's traditional mission of protecting family members of workers will not be maintained. The purpose of this article is to call attention to the implications of changes in the structure of families for Social Security protection.

In what follows, after reporting on the changes in the family structure, we point out the implications of these changes for the auxiliary benefits Social Security offers. After highlighting minorities, older women in poverty, and cohabitation, we conclude by calling attention to some caveats in considering policy proposals.

CHANGING FAMILY STRUCTURE

Dramatic changes in social conventions have occurred during the last 30 years.[1] More and more women have entered the paid labor force. Fewer people marry, they marry later, they divorce more often and sooner, and they also remarry less often. Increasingly many more are not marrying at all. Unmarried-couple households of opposite sex have grown greatly, and cohabiting adults of the same sex have increased their ranks. Summarized here are some important changes:

- Labor force participation rates among women have grown substantially. Among the 24-34 age group, the rate in 1996 was 75 percent, up from 45 percent in 1970. For those age 35-44, 1996's rate of 77.5 percent contrasted with 51.1 percent in 1970. Even for the age group 45-54, traditionally with the highest rate, 1996's rate of 75.4 percent was still considerably higher than 1970's rate of 54.4 percent.
- The median age at first marriage is now 25 years for women and 27 years for men, nearly 4 years later than in 1970.
- Today, only 56% of the adult population (defined as age 18 and over) are married, down from 68% in 1970.
- Families have become smaller. The average family size is 3.19 now, down from 3.58 in 1970.
- Reflecting delayed marriage and later child-bearing, now slightly less than 47% of the married couples have children under 18 living with them, down from 57% in 1970.

- Not only have people been marrying later, more marriages have dissolved. Now, 10% of adults (19 million) are currently divorced, up from 3% (4.3 million) of adults who were divorced in 1970.
- People have also been divorcing sooner and remarrying less. For example, in 1990, among women 25 to 29 who ended a first marriage in divorce, half of them happened in less than 3.4 years, 8 months sooner than 10 years earlier. The remarriage rate after first divorce and the remarriage rate after redivorce have both declined.
- The number of unmarried adults has more than doubled–from 38 million in 1970 to 77 million in 1996.
- The number of never-married adults has also more than doubled–from 21.4 million (16% of all adults) in 1970 to 44.9 million (23% of all adults) in 1996.
- Related to the never-married status, unmarried-couple households of opposite sex have increased more than 7 times–from 523,000 in 1970 to 4 million in 1996. In addition, there are approximately one and one-half million same-sex unmarried couples.

FAMILY STRUCTURE AND AUXILIARY BENEFITS

These long-term trends hold some important policy implications. The central question is who will receive less or no protection if Social Security's benefit provisions for the family are not changed in response.

The family structure changes enumerated earlier have already begun to be reflected in the numbers of new awards for auxiliary beneficiaries in recent years. For example, the proportions of new auxiliary beneficiaries in the total number of new beneficiaries have declined. In 1970, a little more than 54% of new awards went to dependents and survivors. That percentage has steadily declined–to slightly over 40% in 1997, and is estimated to drop further to 35% in 2010 (Table 1).

Several reasons may account for these declines. For example, fewer wife/husband beneficiaries may have resulted from more women receiving benefits as retired workers rather than as wives. The 1981 Social Security Amendments which eliminated benefits to in-school children above age 18 would be a major reason for fewer child beneficiaries. Improved mortality may have reduced the number of survivors.

However, if not legally married, one will not have an eligible spouse or leave an eligible widow or widower, despite a long-term marriage-like relationship. Unless the marriage has lasted for at least 10 years, no one will be eligible for a spouse or survivor benefit when di-

TABLE 1. Proportions of New Beneficiaries[1] as Retired Workers, Disabled Workers, and Dependents and Survivors,[2] in Selected Years, 1970-2010

Year[3]	Retired Workers	Disabled Workers	Dependents and Survivors	Total
1970	36.2%	9.5%	54.3%	100%
1980	38.3	9.4	52.3	100
1990	44.8	12.6	42.6	100
1997	44.5	15.2	40.4	100
2010	48.2	16.7	35.1	100

Notes: [1] New beneficiaries refer to those awarded benefits in each year.
[2] Dependents and survivors include wives/husbands, children, widow(er)s, widowed mothers/fathers and parents.
[3] For 1970-1997, from actual data; for 2010, based on estimates.

Sources: (1) For 1970-1997, calculations based on data in Table 6.A (OASDI Benefits Awarded: Summary), 1998 Annual Statistical Supplement to the Social Security Bulletin, Social Security Administration, SSA Publication No. 13-11700, p. 254.
(2) For 2010, calculations based on unpublished estimates supplied by the Office of the Chief Actuary, Social Security Administration, January 21, 1999.

vorced, except for common-law marriages that are recognized by one of the States.

Beyond the divorced and never-marrieds who are ineligible for these benefits, the problem of lower benefits arises for some beneficiaries, notably widows/widowers. Under current law, a surviving elderly spouse may receive his/her own "retired worker" benefit or a "survivor benefit" based on the deceased spouse's earnings, whichever is higher, but not both. Suppose the husband's retired worker benefit is $1,000/month. If his wife has not worked at all or if her own earnings entitle her to a retired worker benefit of less than $500, then she receives a spousal benefit of $500, half her husband's benefit. Together they receive $1,500. When he dies, she receives $1,000, which is two-thirds their combined benefit. A survivor may do worse than that–getting only half, instead of two-thirds, their combined benefit if husband and wife are each entitled to the same retired worker benefit, say, $1,000. They receive $2,000 between them. When he dies, her benefit stays at $1,000.

These reduced benefits may drive some widows/widowers into poverty, since the official poverty threshold for one elderly person is almost 80% of that for an elderly two-person household. Together with ineligibility, lowered benefits for survivors may help explain (among other reasons) why the poverty rate among nonmarried older women (widowed, divorced, and never married) is now about 20%, four times the rate for older married women.

Changing family patterns may also adversely affect child benefits. Owing mainly to births to unmarried mothers and high divorce rates, 24% of children now live with mothers only. Because women generally earn less than men, child benefits will be lower when they are based on mothers' earnings rather than fathers', unless when paternity is established.

CHANGING FAMILY STRUCTURE AMONG MINORITIES

Further, problems caused by ineligibility and lower Social Security benefits, pointed out above, impact blacks and Hispanics more severely. This is because some of the changes in family patterns have been more pronounced among blacks and Hispanics than whites.[2] An example is the declining percentages of married adults (1970-1996): Whereas the drop was 14% for whites, it was 34% for blacks and 19% for Hispanics. More specifically, the trends for whites, blacks, and Hispanics from 1970 to 1996 are:

1. 14% drop among whites, from 73% to 63%.
2. 34% drop among blacks, from 64% to 42%.
3. 19% drop among Hispanics, from 72% to 58%.

Another example is the increase in never-married persons (1970-1996): 31% increase among whites, compared to 86% increase among blacks and 58% among Hispanics. More specifically, the trends for whites, blacks, and Hispanics from 1970 to 1996 are:

1. 31% increase (from 16% to 21%) for whites.
2. 86% increase (from 21% to 39%) for blacks.
3. 58% increase (from 19% to 30%) for Hispanics.

Still another example is the much larger percentages of their children living with single mothers. Respective percentages for such black, Hispanic, and white children were 51%, 27%, and 18% in 1998.

These trends have resulted in relatively fewer Social Security beneficiaries as dependents and survivors for blacks and Hispanics, compared to whites. The racial/ethnicity dimension is therefore highly significant.

Social Security must adapt to changing family patterns or it will leave behind more and more vulnerable groups of people, many of whom would be black and Hispanic women and children. Future relative declines in auxiliary beneficiaries will be much greater because family pattern changes will affect Social Security recipients with a time lag of decades before changes in family structure result in eligibility or ineligibility for Social Security benefits.

OLDER WOMEN IN POVERTY AND POLICY IDEAS

How women fare under Social Security has become a major issue, with older women in poverty as the predominant concern.[3] The poverty rate for women 65 and over was 13.1 percent in 1997. The differing rates according to marital status were:[4] Married, 4.6%; Widowed, 18.0%; Divorced, 22.2%; Never married, 20.0%. Several ideas have been suggested to deal with the problem: Raise the survivor benefit; raise the survivor benefit and lower the spousal benefit; grant "motherhood credit"; lower the years of marriage requirement; and implement earnings sharing.

COHABITATION

The preceding ideas have been suggested to deal with auxiliary benefits originating from marriages. What about cohabitation which introduces a broader set of circumstances?

Many long-term relationships exist between unmarried partners of the opposite sex. These relationships have grown seven-fold since 1970. Recognition of common-law marriage may ameliorate the situation. But only 12 states in 1999 recognized such marriages, down from 21 states in 1991. Then there is the situation of cohabiting individuals of the same sex. Although statistics are not firm, there is little doubt that the number has increased a good deal in recent years.

Some state and local governmental units and some business firms have recognized domestic partners in granting coverage for health insurance, for example. Some state and local government pension plans allow their participants to designate beneficiaries as they choose. These practices are possibilities. It is also possible to deal with cohabiting situations by means of individual accounts.

CAVEATS IN CONSIDERING POLICY PROPOSALS

In thinking about how to protect at-risk populations, one needs to be mindful of the nature and purpose of the Social Security program. If Social Security is an employment-based income replacement system financed exclusively or largely by the payroll tax, then there is a limit as to what type of benefit (and at what level) would be appropriate.

While it is true that many elderly widows, widowers, and divorcees are disproportionately in poverty, the most important reasons for the income differentials between single and married elderly lie outside the Social Security system. For example, some private pension benefits cease to exist when the retired worker, usually a male, dies. Even if the pension continues for survivors, its purchasing power falls because no private pension is automatically fully adjusted for inflation. In addition, investment income declines as the principal is liquidated to pay for living expenses and health care costs. Is Social Security the appropriate instrument for compensating for the deficiencies in employer pension programs? Should we not explore improvements with other policy vehicles?

NOTES

1. Various U.S. Bureau of the Census publications.
2. Various U.S. Bureau of the Census publications.
3. *White House Conference on Social Security: Viewpoints of Participants,* December 1998.
4. Cited in "Women and Social Security," National Economic Council Interagency Working Group on Social Security, October 27, 1998.

Retirement Patterns and Pension Policy: An International Perspective

M. C. "Terry" Hokenstad
Lennarth Johansson

SUMMARY. Population aging and the changing nature of work are re-shaping thinking about retirement in post-industrial society. The future will see less demarcation between the work and retirement phases of life. This will include a growing trend towards partial retirement and flexible retirement. Changes in pension policy will contribute to changing patterns of retirement. Recent U. S. legislation has uncoupled retirement from Social Security. New policy in Sweden provides partial pensions for partial retirement. Other pension policy changes in the European Union also are contributing to the redefinition of retirement in the 21st century. *[Article copies available for a fee from The Haworth Document Delivery Service: 1-800-HAWORTH. E-mail address: <getinfo@haworthpressinc.com> Website: <http://www.HaworthPress.com> © 2001 by The Haworth Press, Inc. All rights reserved.]*

KEYWORDS. Reshaping retirement, Social Security, pension policy

M. C. "Terry" Hokenstad, PhD, ACSW, is The Ralph S. and Dorothy P. Schmitt Professor and Professor for International Health, Mandel School of Applied Social Sciences, Case Western Reserve University, 10900 Euclid Avenue, Cleveland, OH 44106.

Lennarth Johansson, PhD, is on the staff of the Principal Administrative Office, Care of the Elderly, Swedish National Board of Health and Welfare, Socialstyrelsen SE-106 30 Stockholm, Sweden.

[Haworth co-indexing entry note]: "Retirement Patterns and Pension Policy: An International Perspective." Hokenstad, M. C. "Terry," and Lennarth Johansson. Co-published simultaneously in *Social Thought* (The Haworth Press, Inc.) Vol. 20, No. 3/4, 2001, pp. 25-32; and: *Issues in Global Aging* (ed: Frederick L. Ahearn, Jr.) The Haworth Press, Inc., 2001, pp. 25-32. Single or multiple copies of this article are available for a fee from The Haworth Document Delivery Service [1-800-HAWORTH, 9:00 a.m. - 5:00 p.m. (EST). E-mail address: getinfo@haworthpressinc.com].

As we enter a new millennium, no policy challenge is receiving more attention than public pensions. Around the world, pensions are the subject of intense political debate and occasionally policy action. Recent legislation in the United States has eliminated the social security retirement test as a condition for receiving pension benefits. Sweden is now implementing more extensive pension reform including a flexible retirement benefit. The first decade of the 21st century will witness continued controversy and considerable change in the pension policies of many countries.

What are the forces driving the "pension crisis"? How are these forces likely to impact on both retirement patterns and pension needs? Can public policy help to modify retirement patterns and thus influence the need for pensions? How are different nations addressing these issues? This article will address the global context of these issues and then specially look at the policy debate and action in the United States and Sweden.

POLICY CHALLENGE: DEMOGRAPHIC CHANGE

Population aging is, of course, a major force impacting on pension policy. Populations are aging and longevity is increasing around the world. Every month, one million people turn 60 years of age. This year, 10 percent of the earth's inhabitants are over 60. Two decades from now, one out of three humans will be 60 or older. Of equal significance is the growth of the 80-plus population. It is the most rapidly growing part of the age quake. Two-thirds of earth's inhabitants who have reached 80 years of age from the creation until now are alive today.

Older people are living longer in their post-retirement years. This increasing length of post-60 life expectancy is coupled with a trend towards earlier retirements. The combination of these factors increases the number of years that any one person is likely to draw a pension. The increased length of pension drawing time, added to the overall growth in the number of pensioners, produces what many call the "pension crisis." More people are receiving pensions for longer periods of time.

Work force changes are a related consequence of demographic forces. Lower fertility rates have resulted in a proportionally small young adult population along with the larger senior population. This pattern of population distribution produces worker shortages in times of economic growth. While making unemployment among young people less of an issue, it makes the supply of workers a major concern. One implication could be social policy that encourages older workers to stay in the labor market longer.

Changing population patterns thus have implications for both financing pensions and filling the labor force. While the latter is not yet a major policy issue in the United States because of substantial rates of immigration, it is of growing concern for the demographically aging societies of Europe. Countries that have reached or exceeded zero population growth eventually face worker shortages. In that time, they need to persuade older workers to continue working at least on a part-time basis. The challenge is to make certain there are a sufficient number of workers to fill the work force as fewer babies are born and more people retire.

POLICY OPPORTUNITY: THE NATURE OF WORK

While populations are aging, societies are changing. Economic, technological and societal change is restructuring the environment in which people live. Part of this change is the nature and patterns of work. In a post-industrial age, intellectual skills are much more important than physical strength for the majority of workers. Rapidly expanding knowledge and variations in the type of skill needed increase the likelihood of career change. There is less stability in the world of work, but also greater opportunity for part-time and flexible employment.

Changing patterns of communication are a particular force in shaping new patterns of work. Computer technology and other sophisticated telecommunications systems are resulting in a decentralization of the workplace. More people have their own homes as their place of work. Networks of co-workers are becoming more significant than a street address in many organizations. Geographical decentralization is coupled with the exchange of information and ideas through e-mail and teleconferencing.

Workplace flexibility takes many forms. Project teams are a better way to get things done than reliance on hierarchical structure. Organizational adaptation to the accelerating pace of change requires quicker decision-making and therefore, less hierarchy. The move to increase flexibility also is resulting in an increased reliance on temporary or short-term workers. There is less security in today's workplace for most workers. At the same time, there is increased variety and opportunity for job satisfaction related to the nature of the work.

POLICY REALITY: RESHAPING RETIREMENT

Both the demographic challenge and the changing nature of work are currently reshaping thinking about retirement. Funding concerns in pension policy are largely a result of demographic change. Aging societies face increasing pension costs. Fewer workers pay taxes to support a growing number of pensioners. At the same time, the changing nature of work could lead to greater job satisfaction and therefore happier workers less anxious to retire early. Coupled with the need for older people to remain in an employment-tight labor market, these forces are likely to result in a reshaping of retirement early in this century.

Changing attitudes about retirement are already evident in the "soon to be retired" generation. A recent survey of Baby Boomers by the AARP found the 80% plan to work at least part time after they formally retire. The reasons given varied, but the largest number planned to continue work mainly for the interest or enjoyment that work provides. Other reasons were additional income and starting a new business or a new career. The plans to continue work after "retirement" should not be surprising in spite of current retirement patterns. Self-employed professionals and university professors often work considerably beyond 65 years of age because they enjoy the work they do. Increasing professionalization of the workforce in an information society will, in all likelihood, expand and extend this pattern.

The transformation from an industrial to an information society has implications for all, but certainly for older people. On an individual level it opens the potential of fulfilling both personal and financial goals through a flexible combination of work and leisure. The industrial age life cycle, with its patterns of education in the early years, employment in the middle years and retirement in the later years, is already being modified. Life-long education is an essential part of the post-industrial age. As we have seen, work patterns that are flexible in both time and place are becoming more common. It is no longer necessary to devote full time to work in order to have a job and paycheck.

Retirement remains the part of the life cycle that has been given the least attention. But, it too will be transformed as there is more blending of education, work and leisure. The blended life cycle will produce less demarcation between the gainful employment and non-gainful employment phases of life. A mix of paid work, volunteer participation and leisure time activities will become more common for older people. Terms such as partial retirement and flexible retirement already are widely used by retirement counselors. In fact, many retirement planners now

prefer to be known as "life planners." Clearly retirement is being redefined.

PENSION POLICY: ACTION IN THE UNITED STATES

What impact will these demographic trends and societal forces have
on pension policy? Will public policy itself have any influence on
changing patterns of retirement? Retirement policies and pension programs have been built on an industrial model with the twin goals of providing old age security for seniors and opening up jobs for young
people. These goals, along with the rigor and tedium of the industrial
workplace, have meant that retirement in the early to middle 60's has
been welcome to both the worker and society. In an information society,
neither the nature of work nor the interest of the worker necessitates the
same type of thinking about retirement. Still, seniors do need income
security and public pensions are the most effective poverty prevention
program ever enacted. What are the policy ramifications?

Some are already evident. In addition to fiscal issues, one consideration in public pension reform is to keep older people in the workforce
longer. Policy is being used to keep people working longer into old age
as populations age and the workforce shrinks. Of course, the most obvious way to do this is to increase the age at which a full pension can be received. In the United States, the age for receiving full social security
benefits is being increased from 65 years to 67 years. This change is being instituted over an extended period of time, but there is already political debate over the further extension of the full benefit age to 70. As
one of many proposals put forward to guarantee the long-term fiscal
solvency of the social security system, such pension age proposals, if
enacted, will extend the work life of many workers–particularly those
that can't afford to retire without a full public pension.

Another type of pension reform has just been enacted in the United
States. Recently passed legislation has eliminated the retirement test for
workers 65 years of age and older. This means that workers are now entitled to full social security benefits at age 65 regardless of their current
employment status and the amount of income that they earn from their
jobs. There is no longer a financial penalty for older workers continuing
in the labor market, either full or part time. This policy uncouples retirement from pension policy by no longer limiting pension payments to retired workers.

It is too early to determine the impact of this policy on retirement patterns in the United States. Empirical evidence will be available in a few years. Yet it is safe to assume that the working lives of many Americans will be extended now that there is no longer a financial incentive to retire at 65 years of age. More people will be encouraged to work longer, as the policy will reinforce the transformation of work and promote positive attitudes towards longer working lives. Thus, this pension reform uses the "carrot rather than the stick" approach to keep people working longer.

PENSION POLICY: ACTION IN SWEDEN AND EUROPE

Recent pension reform in Sweden also reflects changing demographics and patterns of work. The new pension policy, which will be fully implemented in 2001, encourages later retirement by basing the amount of the pension on the remaining life expectancy of the pensioner. At the same time, it promotes flexibility in retirement by providing partial pensions for partial retirement any time after age 61. This combination of policy provisions should impact on work as well as retirement patterns in Sweden.

Sweden's pension policy is of particular interest for two reasons. First, Sweden is one of the demographically oldest societies on earth. In fact, it ranked Number One until it was passed by Italy a couple of years ago. Almost 18% of all Swedes are now 65 years of age or older. Low fertility rates and increasing longevity will mean the continued aging of the Swedish population in the future. Thus, it is useful to look at a country that is approximately 20 years ahead of the United States in the aging trajectory.

Also, social and political commitments make old age security and elder care a central feature of an expansive social protection system in Sweden. Its income support and social service programs provide cradle-to-grave security for the Swedish people. Public policy provides the funding and the framework for the provision of programs that have substantially eliminated poverty and reduced the incidence of associated health and human problems. The Swedish pension program is a cornerstone of a health and welfare system that also includes national health insurance, housing allowances and comprehensive home, community and long-term care services for older citizens.

The increasing number of old age pensioners in proportion to the working population has created a challenge to the elder care commitment in Sweden. The increased cost of pension payments is the major reason for pension reform. At the same time, it is considered important to redress inequities in the system. The new pension plan has restructured benefits based on lifetime earnings and linked the pension amount to economic growth.

Another significant change provides pension credits for time devoted to caring for children and for time in post-secondary education. This provision gives more than "lip service" to the importance of parenting. Pension entitlement is received for stay-at-home childcare during the first four years of the child's life. While childcare at home can be credited to the pension account of either parent, it is likely to go most often to the mother's account. This will promote gender equity in pension payments–a progressive step in pension reform. Pension entitlement for study recognizes the value of a well-educated workforce to the society.

All of these areas of pension reform are important, but the inclusion of retirement age flexibility in the reform is particularly significant. Under the new system, pensions are payable in Sweden when a person reaches the age of 61. There is no fixed retirement age and there is nothing to prevent a person from working and receiving a pension at the same time. However, by continuing to work, a worker will increase her or his annual pension in two ways. Pension credits based on salary will increase pension assets and pension credits not used will accumulate for the future. These are incentives for later retirement. The later a person decides to retire, the higher the pension.

In addition to the flexible pension age, the Swedish reform provides flexibility in the amount of pension taken. The pension can be drawn in full or in fractions of one-quarter, one-half or three-quarters of full pension any time from age 61 to age 70. At the latter age, a full pension must be drawn. These options of partial pensions offer flexibility in retirement planning and quite likely will have an impact on retirement patterns after the reform is implemented.

The Swedish reform is a good example of the considerable amount of policy action taking place in the countries of the European Union. Member states in general are enacting changes in pension policy to stem the flow of older workers out of the labor market. These include encouraging part-time work rather than full-time employment. Austria, Belgium, Denmark, Finland, France, Germany, Italy and the Netherlands have all taken some action. This is resulting in the growth of part-time working among both female and male older workers.

European countries still have mandatory retirement ages (either 65 or 67) which serves as an obstacle to flexible retirement. In this area, policy in the United States makes it possible for people to stay in the workforce longer. Demographically-aging Europe must face this issue in the debate around retirement policy.

On the other hand, the United States could well benefit from incorporating a partial pension provision into social security. Partial Social Security payments at an earlier age, coupled with the higher payments the pensioner now receives if retirement is delayed until 70, would be another incentive for later retirement. The increased flexibility also would benefit different types of workers in differing work situations.

CONCLUSION

It is clear that retirement is being redefined in the 21st Century. Both population aging and patterns of work are driving this change. The idea that retirement is a distinct phase devoted to leisure at the end of life is being challenged by changes in the nature of employment as well as pressures on the pension system. Policy makers in a number of countries are recognizing the necessity of pension reform to meet this challenge. Decoupling pensions from retirement and increasing the flexibility of pensions through partial pension programs are two important areas of reform.

Policies increasing the opportunity for older people to play more active economic roles can have a positive impact on the society and the individual. More flexible labor market participation will enable seniors to create a better blend of work, volunteer and leisure time activities in their lives. At the same time, they will be more productive members of the society. We need a strategy to promote productive aging for the sake of the individuals involved and for the sake of the society.

Who Is Responsible
for the Care of the Elderly?
A Comparison of Policies in the United States,
the United Kingdom, and Israel

Carole Cox

SUMMARY. One of the most pressing issues in our society is that of deciding who is responsible for the care of the dependent elderly and how this responsibility should be shared among individuals, families, and government. Both the United Kingdom and Israel have developed policies which focus on community care and that recognize and support the roles of families as caregivers. By examining their systems, valuable insights may be learned that may contribute to the development of policies in the United States. *[Article copies available for a fee from The Haworth Document Delivery Service: 1-800-HAWORTH. E-mail address: <getinfo@haworthpressinc.com> Website: <http://www.HaworthPress.com> © 2001 by The Haworth Press, Inc. All rights reserved.]*

KEYWORDS. Caregiving, informal and formal supports, government, family

INTRODUCTION

It is estimated that by the year 2030 the nursing home population will be 5.3 million, and 13.8 million elderly in the community will need help

Carole Cox, PhD, is Associate Professor, Graduate School of Social Service, Fordham University, 113 W. 60th Street, New York, NY 10023.

[Haworth co-indexing entry note]: "Who Is Responsible for the Care of the Elderly? A Comparison of Policies in the United States, the United Kingdom, and Israel." Cox, Carole. Co-published simultaneously in *Social Thought* (The Haworth Press, Inc.) Vol. 20, No. 3/4, 2001, pp. 33-45; and: *Issues in Global Aging* (ed: Frederick L. Ahearn, Jr.) The Haworth Press, Inc., 2001, pp. 33-45. Single or multiple copies of this article are available for a fee from The Haworth Document Delivery Service [1-800-HAWORTH, 9:00 a.m. - 5:00 p.m. (EST). E-mail address: getinfo@haworthpressinc.com].

with the activities of daily living (U.S. Bipartisan Commission, 1990). Although advances in health care may reduce the likelihood of developing certain illnesses among the elderly, the projected increase in life expectancy will lead to more years spent disabled prior to death (Guralnik, 1991).

There is no more pressing issue in our society than that of deciding how to provide care for the dependent elderly, those persons who are unable to care for themselves. As the size and demands of this population increase, assuring that resources are available to meet their needs is essential. Consequently, a major issue that must be resolved is determining who is responsible for these resources and thus for the care of these dependent persons. Making this decision necessitates an understanding of the roles and expectations of individuals, families, and society with regards to these needs and how they should be addressed.

The decision itself confronts the basic moral tenets of American society as it deals with the issues of social justice, of helping the less fortunate, and the intrinsic worth of the individual. These values become juxtaposed with other salient ones such as personal responsibility, autonomy and rugged individualism. While the former advocate for a system in which society would attend to the needs of those unable to care for themselves, an emphasis on individualism and personal responsibility convey a system in which society and its institutions play only a minor role in meeting these needs.

The dichotomy between these values and beliefs is clearly reflected in the ambiguity and gaps in our long term care policy, that which focuses on issues associated with the care of the chronically ill and disabled, a majority of whom are elderly. Are these persons responsible for their own well-being, are they the responsibility of their families, and how, if at all, should society be involved? What rights and expectations should persons have for care and how and by whom should this care be offered?

As these questions remain unanswered, policy makers struggle with the underlying question of the economics of care provision, particularly the rationing of resources and services and who should receive assistance and how much to offer. While these issues remain unanswered, the nature of future provisions for the elderly requiring assistance remain uncertain. At the same time, answers to these questions are sorely needed as demands for assistance can be expected to increase.

DESCRIPTION OF THE DEPENDENT ELDERLY

Aging is not synonymous with illness or incapacity, but it is associated with expanding rates of dependency. These dependencies result primarily from chronic illnesses that are more common among older persons. Although chronicity itself does not imply frailty, impairments increase with the number of conditions, and older individuals are those most likely to have multiple chronic illnesses (Gurainik et al., 1989). The need for assistance increases dramatically with age. Whereas only 5.9 percent of all persons in the community 65 to 68 have difficulty with one activity of daily living necessary for independence, the proportion increases to 38 percent of those 85 and older (Leon and Lair, 1991).

On the individual level, the burden of dependency is primarily felt through its restrictions on functioning and the potential loss of independence with persons requiring assistance with the basic tasks of daily living. If this assistance is not available in their homes, they must turn to others for such care. For most, the first and primary source of assistance is the family.

THE ROLE OF THE FAMILY AS CARE PROVIDERS

The importance of the family as caregivers to the frail elderly cannot be overestimated. A 1996 nationwide survey to identify and profile the experiences of caregiving indicated that nearly one in four U.S. households contained at least one person acting as caregiver of a relative or friend at least 50 years old (National Alliance for Caregiving and American Association for Retired Persons, 1997). In the 12-month period of the study, 22.4 million households were involved in caregiving. On average these persons spent 15 hours per week caregiving with almost one-fifth providing care for 40 or more hours per week.

When available, the primary caregiver for a frail older person is the spouse with wives constituting 23 percent and husbands 13 percent of all caregivers (Stone, Cafferata, and Sangl, 1987). As a group, these caregivers are likely to be older, to report poorer health, and to receive less assistance, both formal and informal. Frequently, they themselves suffer from chronic illnesses that limit their own activities. However, they are often reluctant to admit to such limitations as this could compromise their ability to provide care and threaten their ability to maintain the person at home.

Spouses care for the frailest elderly, and as they share the same household, they provide extensive levels of assistance (Montgomery and Borgatta, 1989). Moreover, they are likely to have been gradually increasing the amount of assistance they provide and to have been providing some help for long periods. As the frail individual's needs evolve, the spouse is most readily available to attend to them. In fact, it is very common for these needs to be hidden from other members of the family as the couple continues to focus on their independence. The help provided by other family members is generally supplemental to the basic care provided by the spouse (Johnson, 1983).

When further care is required, it is usually the daughter or daughter-in-law who is called upon. The involvement of sons mainly occurs when there is no female sibling to provide assistance. In general, their support tends to be less extensive than the support provided by daughters (Horowitz, 1985). Men tend to provide occasional household help, transportation and assistance with finances while women are involved with the daily household chores, personal care, meal preparation, shopping, and errands (Montgomery and Kamo, 1987; Stoller, 1990).

However, caregiving is not an easy task. Depression, stress, and anxiety have been noted in many studies as frequent symptoms among caregivers (Haley et al., 1987; Cox and Monk, 1996; Schulz et al., 1995). Various factors, dementia, a need for constant supervision, behavior problems, and incontinence exacerbate the strains encountered by caregivers. For many, caregiving occurs at the time of life when they are faced with major work and family responsibilities. Juggling their caregiving roles with their own personal needs, demands and responsibilities is a further source of stress.

The important and major roles played by the family must not be underestimated. As well as offering intimate and consistent support to the dependent elderly, they also relieve the economic burden on the public sector. Data from the National Alliance of Caregivers and the American Association of Retired Persons (NAC/AARP) have been used to develop a national estimate of the economic value of informal care (Arno et al., 1999). Using a market wage approach and a single wage rate, three estimates–low, mid-range, and high–of the value of informal care were developed. Based on 17.9 weekly hours of care at $8.18 hourly wage and 25.8 million caregivers, the mid-range national estimate of the economic value of informal care in 1997 was $196 billion. In comparison to available national spending for home care ($32 billion), nursing home care ($83 billion), and total health care ($1,092 billion), the economic value of informal care is equivalent to approximately 18% of national health care spending and exceeds spending for home care and nursing home care combined.

THE ROLE OF FORMAL SERVICES

The United States

Formal services are used by relatively few caregivers and care recipients. Data from the Supplement on Aging to the National Health Interview Survey and the 1982 Long Term Care Survey indicate that only small proportions, 9% and 5% respectively, receive all of the care from formal providers (Doty, 1986). Moreover, the government finances only a quarter of community care with the remainder paid for by the older persons themselves and their families.

Given the cost of formal services, the reluctance of families to use them is not surprising. Home care costs an average of $75 per visit (National Association for Home Care, 1999) while nursing homes average $56,000 per year (HCFA, 2000). Programs such as respite and day care can be equally expensive, and when available under state-funded or Older Americans Act, generally have long waiting lists. Finally, assistance under Medicaid is primarily focused on those with the lowest incomes, meaning that the middle income families are ineligible for the programs. Consequently, even when caregivers seek assistance, they often find that it is inaccessible.

A major concern in the development of formal services has been that by increasing their availability, families would begin to withdraw their support. Consequently, the public sector would become responsible for the majority of care. However, data continue to show that this does not occur and that families continue to provide assistance to their relatives. A statewide study of service use in Massachusetts found that any substitution of formal for informal services was temporary and related to the availability of the primary caregiver. Even with formal publicly funded home care available, the caregivers used such service only when essential (Tennstedt et al., 1993).

A recent review of the findings from the 1982, 1989, and 1994 National Long Term Care Surveys underscores the lack of helper substitution. Although the use of paid help increased over the survey years, informal caregivers did not decrease their assistance (Liu et al., 2000). Consequently, there is no evidence that the expansion of services does not decrease family involvement or affect the major roles that they assume in providing care for their relatives.

However, the government has been notably absent in its support or assistance to families. The Family and Medical Leave Act of 1993 gives some recognition to their roles by requiring that employers of 50 or more workers offer up to 12 weeks of unpaid leave to an employee to care for a baby, after an adoption, or to provide care for a seriously ill parent, spouse or child. The very restrictions of the Act and the vagueness of many of its terms suggest an underlying ambiguity that can affect its implementation. Moreover, the restricted time limits as well as the necessary size of the employer make the Act meaningless to many caregivers.

As the nation wrestles with the roles of the family and the public sector in providing care to the dependent elderly, much may be learned from the experiences of other countries dealing with the same concern. The United Kingdom and Israel have developed extensive systems of care that focus on meeting the needs of older persons in the community rather than in institutions. Both humanitarian and economic factors have led to the emphasis on home and community based care. Moreover, in each there is a basic recognition of the roles of the family as primary supports and the need for the public sector to supplement them by sharing the responsibility for care.

The United Kingdom

The United Kingdom established its current policies for the care of the elderly with the National Health Services and Community Care Act of 1990 implemented in 1993. This policy focuses on providing care in the community rather than institutions with the local authorities or social service departments responsible for the programs. Primary responsibility for the funding of services shifted to the local governments with some assistance through grants from the central government. The explicit goals of the reforms were:

- to target home-based services on those with the greatest needs so as to enable them to live as normal life as possible in their own homes,
- to ensure that practical assistance for carers is given a high priority in recognition of their own needs for help and support in order to carry out their roles,

- to develop care management so that packages of care are designed in line with individual needs and circumstances.

The local social service departments assume the costs of community services with funding coming from special grants allocated by the central government, local taxes, and client charges. However, people cannot be denied services if they refuse to pay. Eligibility for services is dependent upon assessed need with priority given to the most frail who at the greatest risk of entering an institution.

Under the new community care, caregivers of the older person were to be involved in the assessment and in the development of a care plan. The importance of this was underscored by the following statement of the Minister of Health: "Although not enshrined in legislation, the roles of caregivers most clearly will be given the priority they deserve in all our guidance about assessment, about community care plans, and about all aspects of these proposals" (Bottomley, 1990).

However, as these caregiver assessments were not required, early studies indicated that they were often not conducted. Shortly after initiation of the reforms, a survey of caregivers found little actual improvement in their circumstances (Warner, 1994). If fact, many caregivers reported that services deteriorated and others stated they became more expensive with the new legislation. Only a minority felt that social services had become more attentive to their needs. Many of those surveyed reported that they had not received an assessment and over half did not know about the assessment process. In a further study, Warner (1995) found that nearly half of the social service departments did not assess the needs of the caregivers and those who did receive assessments were less satisfied than they had been in 1993.

Subsequent legislation focused on underscoring and strengthening the roles of family caregivers. The Carers Recognition and Services Act of 1996 gives carers the right to request their own assessment based on their own needs. As the Act emphasizes the importance of these persons in maintaining the elderly and the disabled in the community and the needs they may have for assistance, it remains a landmark piece of legislation with regards to community care.

Evidence suggests that caregivers may now be receiving more attention in the care plan process. In a study of 492 users and carers, almost 90% of the caregivers said they were involved in the assessment process and satisfied with the care packages (Personal Social Services Research Unit, 1998). However, concerns remain that as resources become more restricted, the ability for caregivers to receive services based on their own needs will become limited. Services will be increasingly targeted on the most frail.

Care management plays a pivotal role in community care. Care managers have responsibility for making assessments and formulating appropriate care plans. In doing this they are able to purchase services from the private sector as well as offer public services. The intention is that plans and services are flexible and developed according to the needs of the person. However, as demands for assistance exceed resources, the tendency is to offer assistance based on available services.

Israel

Policy towards the frail elderly in Israel also recognizes the role of the family as the main supports in community care. In 1986, concern over the rising costs of institutional care and the inadequacy of existing community services led to the enactment of the Community Long Term Care Insurance Law (CLTCI). The intent of the Law was to assure alternatives to costly institutionalization by providing for a basket of services that could meet the needs of persons in their own homes. The Law also sought to relieve the burden on the family who provided the majority of care to the frail by supplementing their support with formal services.

Eligibility for services is dependent upon age, the severity of disability, and income. However, the income criterion is set so that only a minority become ineligible for benefits. The Law provides these benefits as part of a social insurance scheme with persons being taxed through their work for the benefits they may need in later years.

The level of functioning is assessed and scored according to a point system with additional points given to those living alone, those with dementia, and those requiring constant supervision. The assessment focuses on a person's ability to perform the ADLs (Activities of Daily Living). The family is not required to be included in the assessment although their involvement is usually recorded. The Law intends to supplement rather than replace family care. Consequently, the family is expected to maintain a significant role in meeting the needs of the older person.

Research findings on the impact of services on the family suggest that their involvement does continue after formal services are introduced. In fact, as indicated in one study (Brodsky and Naon, 1993), caregivers increased their hours of assistance after implementation of the Law. Prior to CLTCI, they had spent an average of 20-21 hours a week in caregiving with this number increasing by two hours after services were initiated. At the same time, even with these increased hours, caregivers reported feeling less stressed. This finding is particularly noteworthy in that it suggests that it is not the hours of care but perhaps the responsibility or the demands associated with particular types of care that are most stressful to caregivers. Having many of the tasks taken over by home care workers may relieve much of the burden on the informal supports.

It is important to recognize that the benefits tend to cover only a small portion of the needs of the dependent elderly, providing a maximum of approximately 18 hours of home care a week for the most disabled. These hours may be complemented with day care and other services such as emergency response systems, meals, and senior centers. In addition, respite centers are available to provide temporary care for periods of three to four weeks as a further measure to relieve the family caregiver.

Community care is also provided to the less disabled low-income elderly through the Ministry of Labor and Social Affairs. Eligibility for these services is determined by income with persons receiving only a pension and a supplement automatically entitled to services. Those receiving services are persons who are generally less disabled than those receiving care under the CLTCI are. Most require some limited assistance or have mobility problems. Among the services provided are home care, day care, meals, and social clubs.

Comparable to the United Kingdom, case managers play major roles in community care for the frail elderly. A nurse or social worker makes the initial assessments for care in the person's home. A panel composed of representatives from the Insurance fund, clinic nurse, and social worker review these assessments. This panel formulates the care plan and selects the care manager. The committee must approve any changes in the plan. The manager is expected to provide regular monitoring and periodic reassessments. However, as caseloads tend to be very large, both monitoring and assessments may be very sporadic. Thus, once services begin, without a major change in the status of the person, they are likely to remain constant.

DISCUSSION

Countries develop policies and programs according to their own cultures, traditions, and values. Thus, what is appropriate and viable in one may not be applicable to another. On the other hand, examining the ways in which others attempt to deal with the pressing problem of a rapidly aging population can provide important insights for policy development in the United States.

The experiences of both the United Kingdom and Israel illustrate the ways in which responsibility for the dependent elderly is being dispersed among families and the government. In both countries, there is a distinct emphasis on community rather than institutional care and recognition of the major roles played by informal caregivers in supporting these persons in their homes. Both have policies that share this responsibility through programs that strengthen or augment the services provided by the family.

In both the United Kingdom and Israel, policies support a multitude of services and programs available on functional need rather than income status. As these services are perceived as entitlements, available to all without a means test, there are no stigmas attached to their use. In both countries, there is the shared assumption that the family is involved and that formal services will not usurp their sense of responsibility.

Certainly, the programs have problems, mostly with regards to budgets and the burgeoning needs of an expanding older population. Assuring adequate resources for services remains a challenge. Possible responses entail raising taxes, increasing the insurance tax, imposing greater charges, or further targeting the services. However, as both Israel and the United Kingdom grapple with these decisions, they do so with strong commitments to community care and to the government's role in its provision.

The United States has yet to clearly define its role and level of responsibility in the support of older frail and disabled persons and their families. Individuals confronting the maze of services, complete with its gaps and inadequacies, that constitute the formal long term care system are generally shocked and dismayed over the cost of services, the strict eligibility requirements of Medicare and Medicaid, and a general absence of accessible programs.

Although services for the frail elderly and their families have continued to develop, access for most remains limited. Medicaid remains the major provider of public service provision for the elderly. However, this dominance is most notable in its support of institutional care. Medicaid finances 48% of all nursing home payments (Levit et al., 1997). Its involvement in home care is considerably less, covering only 14% of home care expenditures in 1996 (Levit et al., 1997). Even when available, Medicaid supported home care, day care, and assisted living tend to have long waiting lists or offer very limited assistance.

Moreover, eligibility for Medicaid is determined by strict income and asset regulations although most states automatically cover those over 65 who receive Supplemental Security Income. However, in order to receive this assistance, persons are commonly forced to impoverish themselves. At the same time, the stigma associated with the program and the impoverished status it requires also means that many who would be eligible do not apply.

Restrictions on Medicare home health visits resulting from the 1997 Balanced Budget Act further limit services to the frail elderly. Although providing basic health care for older persons, the program remains focused on acute care. Thus, in order to qualify for home care the person must be in need of intermittent skilled nursing care or therapy. The program does little to address the needs of the chronically dependent elderly or their caregivers. With patients being discharged earlier from hospitals, families must frequently assume immediately intense caregiving tasks for which they are ill prepared. However, without some formal assistance, their ability to provide this care and to continue in the caregiving role may be severely jeopardized.

It is important to note that whereas the federal government has been slow in its response to the needs of the frail elderly, many states, realizing the mounting costs of nursing home care, have begun to assume greater responsibility. A survey of 25 states found that most of these programs are funded through general revenue funds. The primary services offered are respite care and four or more other services, including information and referral, family consultation or care planning, support groups, care management, and education and training (Coleman, 2000).

Eligibility criteria for these state programs vary although most ignore financial status and use a sliding fee scale or some cost-sharing mechanism to determine fees. However, as many of the programs have very limited budgets, they are able to serve only a small number of caregivers. Several states, in order to further meet the needs of families, have also instituted cash allowance or tax credit programs as well as requiring employers to offer medical leave for those with caregiving responsibilities. Through these policies, the states may lead the way in long term care reform.

America is on the verge of a crisis with regards to the care of the dependent elderly. While the aged population has increased, families have become smaller, and women have become increasingly involved in the workforce. As these trends continue, family caregivers for the elderly will become a scarce commodity. Consequently, appropriate policies and programs to meet the needs of both the caregivers and their relatives are essential.

As these policies are developed, it may be helpful to view the needs of the dependent elderly and their caregivers along a continuum of assistance. In addition, such help should be dependent upon functional rather than economic status. This would assure that services are offered according to real needs. Such interventions may indeed be cost effective by meeting immediate needs of the caregiver and the older person and thus preventing or deterring further deterioration. As an example, a few hours of home care or respite for the caregiver may be all that is required to prevent nursing home placement. Offering transportation to a meals program or day care facility could further enable many older persons to remain in the community.

At the same time, a humane and just system of care demands that policies and services promote and support independence and dignity by offering a variety of choices and flexibility with respect to services and care settings. Autonomy is reinforced when options are available. Recently, much attention has been given to family values and personal responsibility as cornerstones of social policy. As we enter the new millennium, programs must be formulated which adhere to these concepts as they reinforce the dignity and worth of each person, regardless of age or functional ability.

REFERENCES

Arno, P.S., Levine, C., & Memmott, M.M. (1999). The economic value of informal caregiving. *Health Affairs, 18*(2):182-188.

Bottomley, V. (1990). *Evidence to the social services select committee by the health minister.* London: Her Majesty's Stationery Office.

Brodsky, J. & Naon, D. (1993). Home care services in Israel: Implications of the expansion of home care following implementation of the Community Long-Term Care Insurance Law. *The Journal of Cross-Cultural Gerontology, 8:* 375-390.

Coleman, B. (2000). *Helping the helpers: State-supported services for family caregivers.* Washington: Public Policy Institute, AARP.

Cox, C. & Monk, A. (1996). Strain among caregivers: Comparing the experiences of African American and Hispanic caregivers of Alzheimer's relatives. *International Journal of Aging and Human Development, 43*:93-106.

Doty, P. (1986). Family care of the elderly: The role of public policy. *Milbank Memorial Fund Quarterly, 64,* 34-75.

Guralnik, J.M. (1991). Prospects for the compression of morbidity: The challenge posed by increasing disability in the years prior to death. *Journal of Aging and Health, 3(2):* 138-154.

Guralnik, J.M., LaCroix, A.Z., Everett, D.F., & Kovar, M. (1989). *Aging in the Eighties: The prevalence and comorbidity of chronic disease and its association with disability*. Advance Data, 170. Hyattsville, MD: National Center for Health Statistics.

Haley, W.E., Brown, S.L. & Levine, E.G. (1987). Experimental evaluation of the effectiveness of group intervention for dementia caregivers. *The Gerontologist*, 27(3):376-382.

HCFA. Unpublished data (2000). Personal communication with Helen Lazenby.

Horowitz, A. (1985). Family caregiving to the frail elderly. In M.P. Lawton & G. Maddox (Eds.), *Annual Review of Gerontology and Geriatrics, Vol 5*. New York: Springer.

Johnson, C. (1983). Dyadic family relations and social support. *The Gerontologist*, 2:377-83.

Leon, J. & Lair, T. (1990). *Functional status of the noninstitutionalized elderly estimates of ADL and IADL difficulties, research findings 4* (DHHS Publication No. PHS 90-3462). Rockville: Public Health Service.

Levit, K., Lazenby, H., Braden, B., Cowan, C., Sensenig, A., McDonnell, P., Stiller, J., Won, D., Martin, A., Sivarajan, L., Donham, D., Long, A. & Stewart, M. (1997). National Health Expenditures, 1996. *Health Care Financing Review*, 19:161-200.

Liu, K., Manton, K., & Aragon, C. (2000). *Changes in home care use by older persons with disabilities: 1982-1994*. Washington: AARP.

Montgomery, R. & Borgatta, E. (1989). The effects of alternative support strategies on family caregiving. *The Gerontologist*, 29:457-464.

Montgomery, R. & Kamo, Y. (1987). *Differences between sons and daughters in parental caregiving*. Paper presented at the Annual Meeting of the Gerontological Society of America, November, Washington, DC.

National Alliance for Caregiving and the American Association of Retired Persons. (1997). *Family caregiving in the U.S.: Finding from a national survey*. Bethesda: NID.

National Association for Home Care (1999). *Basic statistics about home care, 1999*. Washington, DC: Author.

Personal Social Services Research Unit (1998). *Evaluating community care for elderly people, 2*. Canterbury: University of Kent.

Schulz, R., O'Brien, A.T., Bookwala, J., & Fleissner, K. (1995). Psychiatric and physical morbidity effects of dementia caregiving: Prevalence, correlates, and causes. *The Gerontologist*, 35(6):771-791.

Stoller, E. (1990). Males as helpers: The role of sons, relatives, and friends. *The Gerontologist*, 30:228-236.

Stone, R., Cafferata, G.L., & Sangl, J. (1987). Caregivers of the frail and elderly: A national profile. *The Gerontologist*, 27:677-683.

Tennstedt, S., Crawford, S., & McKinlay, J. (1993). Is family care on the decline? A longitudinal investigation of the substitution of formal long-term care services for informal care. *The Milbank Quarterly*, 7(4):601-624.

U.S. Bipartisan Commission on Comprehensive Health Care (1990). *A call for action: The Pepper commission final report*. Washington: U.S. Government Printing Office.

Warner, N. (1994). *Community care: Just a fairy tale?* London: Carers National Association.

Warner, N. (1995). *Better tomorrows?* London: Carers National Association.

Pakistan's Zakat System:
A Policy Model for Developing Countries as a Means of Redistributing Income to the Elderly Poor

Grace Clark

SUMMARY. Pakistan's national zakat system is a simple welfare system based on traditional Islamic law. It provides minimal benefits to the very poorest of Pakistan's poor, especially the elderly. Although the system was launched with the highest religious ideals, utilizing creative approaches to collecting and disbursing zakat, over time this system has experienced deficiencies due to corruption, favoritism, and government greed. While zakat has not met the original goals of eliminating poverty or eliminating beggary, and while it has met the goals of providing rehabilitation and redistributing income in only the most modest sense, Pakistan has still demonstrated the potential for a zakat system to provide some cash income to the very poorest old in a very poor country who would otherwise have no cash income at all. *[Article copies available for a fee from The Haworth Document Delivery Service: 1-800-HAWORTH. E-mail address: <getinfo@haworthpressinc.com> Website: <http://www.HaworthPress.com> © 2001 by The Haworth Press, Inc. All rights reserved.]*

Grace Clark is Acting Director of the International Center on Global Aging at the National Catholic School of Social Service of the Catholic University of America, Shahan Hall, Washington, DC 20064.

[Haworth co-indexing entry note]: "Pakistan's Zakat System: A Policy Model for Developing Countries as a Means of Redistributing Income to the Elderly Poor." Clark, Grace. Co-published simultaneously in *Social Thought* (The Haworth Press, Inc.) Vol. 20, No. 3/4, 2001, pp. 47-75; and: *Issues in Global Aging* (ed: Frederick L. Ahearn, Jr.) The Haworth Press, Inc., 2001, pp. 47-75. Single or multiple copies of this article are available for a fee from The Haworth Document Delivery Service [1-800-HAWORTH, 9:00 a.m. - 5:00 p.m. (EST). E-mail address: getinfo@haworthpressinc.com].

47

KEYWORDS. Zakat, elderly, redistribution of income, welfare systems in developing countries, Islamic law, volunteers

INTRODUCTION

The United Nations International Year of the Older Person in 1999 focused attention on the rapidly increasing number of older persons in developing countries. Developed countries have been experiencing a gradual increase in the number and proportion of older people for many years, and they have established pensions and other schemes to provide for the financial needs of their older citizens. In contrast, this is a relatively new phenomenon for most developing countries, many of whom have doubled the number of older persons in the last twenty years and are likely to double or triple the number again in the next twenty-five years (U.S. Census Bureau, 1996). Many of these developing countries do not have either the financial resources or a tax structure that would facilitate setting up either a social security system or a pension system. Most do not have the resources to set up even a simple entitlement welfare system to provide for the needs of poor older persons who cannot earn a living and who do not have family or financial resources to support them.

For developing countries, including most predominantly Muslim countries, increasing numbers of older persons, combined with the impact of modernization and urbanization, has resulted in growing numbers of older people left without a source of income (Belokrenitsky, 1984). Compounding the problem, many developing countries require mandatory retirement at fairly young ages, precluding the possibility that older persons might earn a living to support themselves. Then, too, the majority of people in most developing countries are desperately poor to start with, so that if they lose their income in old age, they have few resources to fall back on. Developing countries need to find models of redistributing income that can help at least the most vulnerable poor elderly in their societies.

In addition to the financial constraints that preclude adopting Western systems, many of these formerly colonial nations find it politically difficult to institute a Western-style pension or social security system. These countries need to find alternatives to Western models, preferably models based on familiar indigenous systems or religious institutions familiar to that country's population.

At the same time that the number of older persons in predominantly Muslim countries has grown rapidly, there has also been a resurgence of Islam, not only as a religion, but also as a political and ideological force. Within the last 40 years, there have been a number of Muslim theorists calling for the reformation of predominantly Muslim states so that their laws and social institutions become more Islamic (Afzul ur-Rahman, 1974; Maududi, 1978; Mannon, 1980; Khurshid Ahmad, 1980).

This article examines one of these new Islamic social policies, Pakistan's national zakat system, as a potential model of an indigenous, familiar social institution that can provide some financial assistance to the very most needy of the elderly poor. Although Pakistan's national zakat system was not designed specifically as a system to provide financial assistance to the elderly poor, over half the recipients of zakat are older widows and sick and frail elderly of both sexes. Zakat is, in reality, a financial system that helps older persons.

Pakistan's national zakat system is an excellent example of a developing country trying to help its most vulnerable citizens by using a system based on traditional Muslim religious practices rather than on models borrowed from first world countries. This case study demonstrates how this system, based in Islamic law, has the potential to serve as a vehicle to redistribute income to the elderly and to achieve a measure of social justice. It also shows that the goals of any social policy, even one based on religious law, can be thwarted in implementation. This study is important because it demonstrates both positive and negative aspects of Pakistan's zakat system at a time when many predominantly Muslim countries are considering such policies.

The author would like to make it clear that this is not an analysis of zakat as a traditional religious duty in Islam. Rather, it is an examination of a policy of the government of Pakistan, which is based on traditional zakat.

THE SITUATION OF OLDER PEOPLE IN PAKISTAN

Pakistan's 1998 Census counted over 130 million people. Pakistanis aged 60 and older comprise 5.5% of the population or 7 million people (Government of Pakistan, 1999). Pakistan is a predominantly agrarian society. The majority of all Pakistanis, including the elderly, live in small villages. Like many developing countries, Pakistan is rapidly undergoing urbanization and modernization, with many families leaving elderly parents behind in its small rural villages.

Pakistan's retirement age is 60, but this applies to only a small number of people, mostly wage earners in large industries, government civil servants, and the military. The presence of a mandatory retirement age, however, along with an enormous and growing number of youth, makes it almost impossible for anyone over 50 to find new paid employment. Then, too, most Pakistanis over 60 are illiterate–60% for men and 90% for women. This makes it very difficult to compete with younger age cohorts who tend to be better educated. Fewer than 10% of women 60 and over are economically active in any capacity.

Pakistan's implicit policy is that the aged will take care of themselves from work, assets, or savings, or, if they cannot do that, then their sons will take care of them. There are no statistically valid studies to support or refute this assumption, although Pakistan's National Council of Social Welfare is currently engaged in a study to address this and other issues relating to older persons.

Pakistani 1998 Census data suggests that between those who never marry, those who have no children, those whose children die before adulthood, and those who have no sons, between 14% to 17% of Pakistan's elderly, or a million elderly, have no adult son who could possibly support them. In addition, while many sons who have migrated to urban areas to work dutifully send money back to aging parents in rural areas, many are too poor to support another person in a separate household. Then, too, in any society, not everyone does what is expected of him. Furthermore, while parental support is a social and moral obligation in Pakistan, it is not a legal obligation, as spousal support is, so that neither the parents nor the state could sue adult sons to require them to support their parents.

Large numbers of Pakistani women over 60 are widows. Because women tend to marry older men, there are more widows than widowers in each age cohort. Additionally, while men often remarry if they lose a spouse, it is unusual for women who have had children to remarry. It is very rare for older widows to remarry. The 1998 Census showed that over 80% of the men over 60 are currently married, while only 50% of the women over 60 are married. This disparity increases markedly with age.

Older women are especially vulnerable financially. For the most part, men in Pakistan control women's lives–first as fathers, then as husbands, and then as sons or other male relatives. This is supported through law, social custom, and economic control. While both Islamic and Pakistani law permit women to inherit, it is common practice for men in her family to manage those assets. A widow is supposed to inherit a one/eighth share of her husband's estate, but it is common for her son to manage this for her along with his own share. A daughter inherits one-half her brother's share, since it is assumed that the brother will have a family to support and is supposed to support his widowed mother. In practice, this means that the men in the family tend to retain control of what resources exist. It is common for older women to have no real control over their own inheritance, much less any other income. Moreover, for the majority of very poor Pakistanis, there is no money to inherit. In several small surveys of older Pakistanis, between 70% and 100% of older women surveyed had no cash income of any kind (Afzul, 1999; Clark and Zaman, 2000; Dar, 1996). This makes widows completely dependent for survival on the good will of others, commonly their sons. If they have no sons or their sons will not support them, widows become dependent on the good will of more distant relatives and neighbors.

Ninety-seven percent of Pakistan's population is Muslim, with about 10 to 15% of these Shia Muslims. Muslims, including Muslims in Pakistan, share the common Abrahamic tradition that includes the Ten Commandments, the fourth of which is, "Honor thy father and thy mother that their days may be long upon the earth." The Quran reinforces this with many injunctions to honor one's parents and support them financially and in other ways. The Quran even maintains that Heaven is at the feet of your mother. Traditional custom also supports the value of supporting one's parents, and, by extension, all older people. While actual practice in relation to supporting parents and other elders may vary, national values support the concept that it is socially just for government to see to the well-being and support of older persons.

BACKGROUND ON ISLAM AND ZAKAT

"Islam" means "submission to God." Islam is a complete way of life that integrates spiritual belief, religious practice, law and society according to the revelations given to the Prophet Mohammed and set down in the Quran, Islam's Holy Book. Followers of Islam are called Muslims. In Islam, each Muslim is equal before God and he or she must answer to God as an individual on the Day of Judgment.

One of the most important concepts in Islam is "Tawhid" or "Unity," especially the Unity of God (Allah) and the Unity of God and His Creation. The concept of unity is also used to reflect the unity of the community of believers. Essential to this unity is the responsibility of each Muslim to the other members of the Muslim community.

Zakat is one of the five "pillars of Islam," behaviors required of Muslims to demonstrate their faith and devotion to Allah (God). (The other requirements are the profession of faith, prayer five times a day, fasting during the holy month of Ramadan, and the pilgrimage to Mecca.) Zakat is the giving of alms to certain groups of people specified in the Quran and Sunnah, the Traditions of the Prophet. These are the poor (no income), the needy (some income, but not enough to meet one's needs), recent converts to Islam, those in debt through circumstances beyond their control, travelers, slaves to be emancipated, those who collect and disburse zakat, and those who do the good works of God (Crane, 1981; Tanzil ur-Rahman, 1981). There are over 100 instances in which the Quran exhorts Muslims to give zakat, particularly emphasizing giving zakat to the poor who are widows and orphans (Siddiqi, 1983). Traditionally, the primary function of zakat has always been as an act of piety for the giver to show his own gratitude for God's blessings. Another important function of zakat is that it reinforces the unity of the Muslim community by reinforcing the responsibility of all Muslims for the poor and vulnerable members of their society (Aghnides, 1981; Maududi, 1978).

In Pakistan, the majority of the population is Sunni Muslim, and most of them follow the Hanafi fiqh, one traditional set of interpretations of Islamic law. Under Hanafi fiqh, zakat is owed once a year during the holy month of Ramadan, although Muslims are encouraged to give zakat at any time. Hanafi fiqh holds that zakat is an absolute gift to the individual recipient for himself (or herself) and his dependents. There should be no strings attached. There are different rates of zakat for different types of assets, but the general rate is 2.5 percent (Maududi, 1978; Qureshi, 1979).

Zakat is payable by those who are "sahib-e-nisab," or "wealthy persons," those who hold income and assets above what one needs to provide for one's family for a year. If one does not have this level of income or assets, one is exempt from the requirement to pay zakat. One is only required to pay zakat if one can afford it (Aghnides, 1981).

Zakat was compulsory during the time of the Prophet and the first four caliphs. During the caliphate of Ali, the payment of zakat became embroiled in the issue of the legitimacy of the government. After Ali's death, his followers, later known as Shias, refused to pay zakat to his successor because they did not recognize the government's legitimacy. Zakat as a government institution ended during the reign of Umar bin Abdul Aziz in Baghdad (717-720 AD). At that time several prominent jurists concluded that Muslims should pay their zakat directly to the poor and that government was prohibited from forcing a Muslim to take an oath about the extent of his assets (Siddiqi, 1983). With a few isolated exceptions over history, zakat has been an individual responsibility, for all practical purposes, since 720 AD.

From the time that Pakistan began as a state in 1947, there have been Islamic theorists who have pressed for Pakistan's policies to be based on Islamic law and tradition. Some, such as Maulana Maududi (1978), belong to a group that Yvonne Haddad (1982) refers to as "ideological engineers" (also Mannon, 1980; Siddiqi, 1983; Qureshi, 1979; Al-Qardiwi, 1981). They believed that a zakat system should be part of an ideal Islamic state that would recreate the Golden Age of Islam. Others posited Islamic economics as an alternative to Western Capitalism or Communism. They see zakat as an Islamic safety net, which helps to redistribute wealth and care for the needs of the poor (Khurshid Ahmad, 1980). While their proposals differed, all of them called for the implementation of zakat as part of a program of economic justice in an Islamic government citing the tradition of the elimination of poverty during the Golden Age of Islam.

Moreover, political events in the 1970's throughout the Islamic world fueled the concept of an Islamic society in which zakat played an important role in achieving economic justice. Zulfikar Ali Bhutto's election victory in the early 1970's was based in part on his vision of an Islamic version of socialism that included the redistribution of wealth. While he nationalized the banks and some heavy industry, Bhutto did not institute a zakat system or a welfare system, and he did nothing to help the elderly poor (Khan, 1981).

In the late 1970's, Pakistan clearly had widely ranging levels of wealth. While some rich and middle class people gave zakat to poor people, it was purely personal, irregular, often based on the donor's relationship to the recipient and on the individual donor's understanding of zakat. A survey done by Sabzwari (1979) in a middle-class subdivision of Karachi found that while 75 percent said that they had heard of zakat, only five percent practiced it themselves. From that and other sources, it appears that, whatever the rhetoric of the late 1970's, the majority of Sunni Muslims in Pakistan did not practice zakat in the traditional way.

INTRODUCTION OF PAKISTAN'S ZAKAT SYSTEM

General Zia ul-Haq seized power on July 5, 1977, establishing a military government and later naming himself as President. In 1978, President Zia asked the Council of Islamic Ideology to explore the concept of a zakat system for Pakistan as part of a series of potential legal changes based on Islamic law (Government of Pakistan, 1980). Based on their encouragement (Tanzil ur-Rahman, 1981), President Zia appointed a task force to develop a plan for a national zakat system in Pakistan, based on the traditional Islamic system.

In 1980, President Zia promulgated the Zakat and Ushr Ordinance of 1980, which forms the legal mandate for Pakistan's national zakat system. In introducing the system, President Zia (1980) called zakat an "essential pillar of Islam's welfare system." The Preamble to the Ordinance states "the prime objection of the collection of zakat, and disbursements therefrom, is to assist the needy, the indigent and the poor." Based on President Zia's introduction and the ordinance itself, the general public expected zakat to have an impact in four ways:

1. It would provide financial assistance to those in need and who could not work.
2. It would provide economic rehabilitation for those who could work.
3. It would eliminate beggary.
4. It would redistribute wealth in the society.

In addition to these goals explicitly stated in the ordinance, discussions in Pakistan in 1983 indicated that most Pakistanis had two additional goals:

5. Some Pakistanis expected the system to eliminate poverty.
6. Most people seemed to feel that the government would be more conscientious about running a program based on important Islamic beliefs.

The Zakat and Ushr Ordinance of 1980 balanced a number of political factors. It appealed to those who wanted to move Pakistan toward becoming an Islamic state. It gave the appearance of redistributing income, thus pleasing the poor and idealists.

How Pakistan's Zakat System Worked Initially

In concept, Pakistan's national zakat system is very simple. Money is collected from the bank accounts of those deemed *sahib-e-nisab*, sent to the central government and distributed through a hierarchical system of administration to a nationwide network of local zakat committees (LZCs) who determine eligibility and are responsible for the disbursement of zakat to the selected mustahaqeen, "worthy poor." The following section provides a brief description of how the system worked for the first several years of its existence.

The zakat law requires that on the first day of the Muslim holy month of Ramadan, banks in Pakistan must deduct 2 and 1/2 percent from all the bank accounts above the *Nisab* amount, which may be adjusted each year to keep pace with inflation. The *Nisab* amount was Rs. 1000 in 1980, Rs. 2000 in 1981 and 1982, and Rs. 3000 in 1983. Non-Muslims and Shias can be exempted from this deduction by filing a form with the bank that says either that they are not Muslim (such as Christians or Hindus), or that they are Muslim, but that government-collected zakat is against their fiqh. Non-Pakistani Muslims can also be exempted. Most money collected by the government for zakat in Pakistan came from Sunni Muslims (Khan).

After deducting the zakat from the accounts, the banks sent the funds directly to the Ministry of Finance. The Zakat and Ushr Ordinance (1980) called for zakat funds to be distributed to the provinces according to each province's percentage of the total population.

The organization of the national system for determining eligibility and disbursing zakat was/is essentially hierarchical, with parallel bodies at the national, provincial, district, tehsil, and local levels. The closer to the top of the organization a level was, the more it was concerned with policy formulation and overall coordination. The closer to the bottom of the organization, the more it was concerned with operations.

The Central Zakat Council (CZC) is the national body responsible for broad policy decisions related to zakat. The Chairman of the CZC is a serving Justice of the Supreme Court of Pakistan. Other members are volunteers, some from the public sector and some religious scholars. Still other members of the CZC are government officials responsible for the implementation of zakat at the national or provincial level. The Central Zakat Council meets quarterly to review the work of the federal and provincial zakat administrations and to make major policy decisions that interpret the implementation of the law.

Initially, Pakistan's national zakat system was administered by the Central Zakat Administration (CZA). These professionally trained civil servants supervised the ongoing administration of the zakat system throughout Pakistan, coordinating the work of approximately 300,000 people in 1983. CZA implemented policy changes originating in law or the decisions of the CZC, and itself made minor policy decisions affecting the collection or disbursement of zakat. It also wrote and updated the zakat administrative manual, kept records, provided training for provincial and district zakat officials, and published a monthly magazine for local zakat committees, *al-Zakat*. It authorized disbursement of zakat to the provinces. In 1983, the CZA managed Pakistan's national zakat system with 14 professional staff.

The national zakat system's first Administrator General Zakat, I. A. Imtiazi, insisted he would only take the position if funds for his salary and other administrative and staff costs were paid out of the consolidated funds budget of Pakistan (i.e., general tax revenues), not the zakat collections. President Zia agreed, and a special fund was established that held only zakat collections. All the disbursements from that fund were only for payments to provinces for eventual distribution to the mustahaqeen. Administrative costs for provincial and other levels of administration came out of provincial consolidated funds, not zakat funds. For the first fifteen years of zakat, the government very carefully kept zakat money in a special fund. It was equally careful about keeping records and reporting to the government, the public, and the LZCs on the total amounts collected and disbursed (Imtiazi, 1999).

In addition to the national level administration, each province had a Provincial Zakat Council (PZC) which modified policy to meet the specific needs of its province, but in congruence with federal policy. An important role for the Provincial Administrator Zakat was to sit on the Central Zakat Council, report on his province, and to advocate policy or administrative decisions that dealt with issues that particularly affected his province. The Provincial Administrator Zakat sat in one of the Provincial ministries, although this varied by province. Provincial Zakat Administrations disbursed zakat funds to District Zakat Committees (DZCs) in proportion to each district's population. Similarly, there were committees based at the district, and, in the beginning, the tehsil levels.

The Local Zakat Committees (LZCs) perform most of the operational work of the zakat system. In 1983, there were 37,033 LZCs throughout Pakistan, each with seven unpaid volunteers, all men. The Chairman of the LZC was supposed to be elected by the other members, although sometimes he was appointed by the local powerbroker. The LZC's primary function was to determine eligibility for zakat, to disburse funds, and to keep records of disbursements and meetings. According to Attar Mahmud, Deputy Administrator Zakat in 1983-84, at least one person on the committee was supposed to be literate, but over one-quarter of all LZCs had no literate member (Clark, 1985). Generally, it was considered an honor to be a member of an LZC.

One of the most important functions of the LZC was determining eligibility for zakat. The *Zakat and Ushr Ordinance of 1980* specified certain groups of people eligible for zakat based on the groups mentioned as eligible in the Quran. These are widows, orphans, the sick and disabled, students, and religious students. (Not all the groups mentioned in the Quran were included in Pakistan's ordinance.)

Most LZCs had no formal written applications. This was seen as unnecessary, since the reason for so many LZCs was so that LZC members would know the personal situations of the poor in their community and could re-evaluate them regularly. Poor persons who thought they were eligible applied to individual LZC members. Other times, members of the LZC nominated people that they knew personally to be poor and needy. Only Muslims were eligible to receive a zakat grant. Although Shias did not contribute zakat to Pakistan's system, as Muslims they were eligible to receive zakat; however, local interpretation by LZCs varied on this issue.

Each LZC considered all of the recommendations for zakat together and made its determinations based on what its members thought was appropriate for the community. When zakat first began, zakat funds were disbursed to each LZC in six-month intervals. LZCs had great discretion in how they would allocate the money, as long as recipients were poor and fit one of the categories specified by the law. Some LZCs gave zakat to all those they considered in need. This diluted the amount any one person received. The LZC was not required to give any grants to any group, although on the whole, elderly widows received a little over half the grants. In 1983-84, the most common amount granted for a monthly stipend was Rs. 100 per month, although some grants provided as little as Rs. 12 (Clark, 1985).

Initially, the LZCs were also authorized to spend the money for economic rehabilitation. The LZCs could also spend the money on health care for a poor person or for dowries for poor orphaned girls to marry. Most rehabilitation grants ranged from Rs. 500 to purchase a sewing machine or small tools to Rs. 5000 for a water buffalo. If the LZC disbursed money for rehabilitation, it came out of its total allocation, so that it had less money to provide living stipends to widows, orphans, and others. Very few funds were ever disbursed to the elderly for economic rehabilitation.

In the early 1980's, recipients were paid in cash directly from the LZC members. The recipient signed his name that he had received the specified amount, or, since the vast majority of the recipients were illiterate, he signed with a thumbprint. Disbursement records were kept in the LZC's record book. LZCs with no literate member were allowed to spend up to Rs. 100 per six-month period for a secretary who was not a member of the LZC.

Clark's survey (1985) of the LZCs as well interviews with over two hundred people both in and out of the zakat system found that no one thought these zakat grants were adequate. Except for one official in Lahore, no one thought the zakat system eliminated poverty. Some did think zakat had helped somewhat to reduce beggary. Most people thought the zakat system had helped a little to alleviate the suffering of some of Pakistan's most vulnerable people, and they were proud of their role in that.

While occasional newspaper stories contained reports of individual LZC members or officials helping themselves to zakat funds, these incidents were rare. Discussions with many members of LZCs and others involved with the system revealed that most felt the Quran specifically required that zakat had to go to poor people. They took very seriously the Quran's teaching that God would be especially harsh in His punishment on the Day of Judgment for anyone who had stolen from widows and orphans. One person quite explicitly stated that he did not mind cheating the government of Pakistan at all, but he believed the Prophet had explicitly forbidden taking zakat money, and he would not risk eternal punishment. Follow-up by the provincial or district officials on reports of inappropriate disbursements usually found the persons receiving zakat were actually eligible, and that that LZC had had many more applicants for zakat who were eligible than the LZC had funds for. In checking the books during visits to LZCs, the author found that several local committees disbursed more than they had received. When asked about this, LZC members of several committees sheepishly explained that they were embarrassed by the small size of the grants that the government had provided. Since their own reputations were on the line in the village, many had quietly supplemented the funds out of their own pockets, although most were not wealthy men.

At the national level, the zakat system was a very straightforward, well-run system. In six months at the Central Zakat Administration, the author had access to records, memoranda, daily conversations, and, after a few months even special reports designed for President Zia's eyes only. Except for the Presidential reports, these records were essentially open to anyone who wanted to read them. Throughout that entire time, everyone at CZA was proud of what he was doing and willing to talk about it. Staff of CZA ranged from the very serious and pious approach of the Administrator Zakat who saw zakat work as a religious duty, to other staff members who saw themselves as good civil servants just trying to do a good job starting a new program with limited resources. There was never any sign that any individual profited personally from zakat in any way. When documented reports came in of anyone mishandling zakat funds, staff at the CZA took quick action to deal with it.

Changes to Zakat Policy Over Time

During the years when Zia was in power, zakat continued as it had started. In 1985 the zakat law was amended to require two members of each LZC to be Muslim women of good character over 45 years of age, increasing the size of LZCs to nine members. Although the original law did not require LZC members to be men, none of the 37,000 LZCs in 1984 had a female member.

After Zia's death, more and more reports surfaced of mismanagement of zakat funds. After Nawaz Shariff became Prime Minister in 1991, he authorized a management evaluation of the zakat system, which was completed that year. Shirazi (1996) cites the report as finding serious mishandling of funds throughout the system. This mishandling included appropriation of zakat funds by LZC members for personal use, kickbacks to zakat committee members, shoddy recordkeeping, in part due to illiteracy, and favoritism in the selection of recipients. The Zakat Administration followed up the report by preparing federal legislation addressing these problems.

The zakat law was changed in 1994 so that recipients no longer received cash in their village. Instead a system of crossed checks was introduced. Each quarter the LZCs sent the DZC a list of zakat recipients. Most districts now limited the number of zakat recipients per LZC to 10. The DZCs deposited Rs. 900 into each recipient's bank account (Rs. 300 for each of three months). Then the LZC wrote each individual recipient a check. The recipient then needed to present the check to the bank in person, signing with a thumbprint, in order to receive the money in her account.

Several problems arose. Most banks required accounts to maintain a minimum balance of Rs. 500. This meant that a recipient's grant for the first quarter under the new system was not really Rs. 900, but Rs. 400. Moreover, most banks also required the recipients to come with the LZC chairman on a certain day of the quarter to withdraw their money. Since many banks are some distance from the villages, this created a further inconvenience. Many recipients depended on the chairman for a ride to the bank. Some chairmen charge for this service, although this is not allowed under the law.

Interviews with LZC members and recipients and feedback from questionnaires document that most people do not like this bank-based system. It is difficult for everyone. And, of course, it is just as possible to cheat this system as the old one. What LZC members point out is that most of them are honest and that this new system just makes life much more difficult for them and the recipients. They say they feel bad requiring old and sick people to travel any distance, especially in summer when it may be extremely hot. One committee even reported that one older woman died from the heat while waiting at the bank for her zakat.

The 1994 law brought other changes. Tehsil Zakat Committees were eliminated. The Central Zakat Administration was moved from the Ministry of Religious Affairs to the Finance Ministry (Qureshi, 1999). Also, the Central Zakat Council established fixed percentage distributions for zakat funds. The rates are as follows:

Subsistence	60%
Education scholarships	18%
Scholarships for religious training schools	8%
Health institutions	6%
Social welfare rehabilitation	4%
Dowries for orphan girls	4%

While this distribution scheme may not at first glance appear to have anything to do with the elderly, the great majority of those receiving the subsistence allowance are the elderly, especially widows. (Others receiving subsistence are young widows with children and handicapped persons.) These legal changes created a sum of money that was theoretically targeted at the very poorest and most vulnerable elderly in Pakistan.

Under the revised law, only money for subsistence and education scholarships is sent to the LZCs. The remaining money is held by the District Zakat Committee and disbursed as money allows on the recommendation of the LZCs. For health expenditures, each hospital has a committee, which includes the chief medical officer and the social worker, among others. They recommend to the DZC which needy persons should receive health treatments to be paid by zakat funds. The DZC makes the final approval on these recommendations. Some of the treatments paid for include quite expensive treatments such as chemotherapy, surgery, and kidney dialysis.

The biggest policy change to the zakat system came in 1995, when the Benazir Bhutto government "centralized" zakat. The 1995 amendments completely bypassed the provincial and district governments. In theory this was supposed to mean the federal government would be responsible not only for the collection of zakat, but also for its disbursement. While the amendments maintained the DZCs and LZCs in principle, in practice, they received no government communications or money. The whole zakat infrastructure was allowed to dissolve.

This policy of "centralization" meant that the federal government collected zakat, but did not disburse it. This change became evident after the collection of zakat in 1995. Zakat was collected but not disbursed to anyone. For the next two collection cycles, zakat was collected, but not disbursed anywhere in Pakistan except for a few cosmetic disbursements in Islamabad.

Moreover, whereas the original zakat system kept zakat funds separate from other funds, beginning in 1995, zakat collections simply became part of the consolidated fund (general fund), along with all other federal government revenue. This made it difficult to determine how much zakat had been collected, and how much and when zakat was disbursed to the provinces. Also, since 1995, the federal government has become very secretive about zakat collections and disbursements.

What is astonishing is that few people realized the magnitude of the failure to disburse zakat funds. Many local people who had been LZC members before 1995 noticed that the mustahaqeen were not receiving any payments, but they assumed that there was some local problem of corruption or bureaucratic delay. Based on reports from some district bank managers who collected zakat, on previous government reports of annual collections, and on conversations with people involved in the renewed zakat system, the author estimates that about Rs. four billion per year were collected but not disbursed in 1995, 1996, and 1997. A senior retired zakat official who asked not to be named corroborated this figure.

In 1997, the new government of Nawaz Sharif restored the legal mandate for the previous system of zakat, and reestablished the provincial, district and local zakat structures. It also changed the process for determining LZC chairs from local elections to appointment by the local member of the National Assembly. Also, the Central Zakat Administration was moved back to the Ministry of Religious Affairs.

Justice Munawar Mirza of the Pakistan Supreme Court, Chairman of the Central Zakat Council from 1997 to 2000, oversaw the rebuilding of the zakat infrastructure. In late 1998, zakat was distributed in Baluchistan and some parts of Punjab. In 1999, zakat was distributed throughout the country. Part of the administrative change under the new administration, however, is that the Central Zakat Administration now only releases half a province's quarterly allotment at a time. It will not release the other half until the province has disbursed more than half of the initial allotment. Given the pipeline nature of any public benefits program, this requirement tends to tie up money and slow down its distribution. The Chair of the Central Zakat Council sees this as being prudent and saving money, but he was unclear what impact this would have on recipients (Mirza, 1999). Moreover, both the Administrator of Zakat and the Chair of the Central Zakat Council stated that there is no plan for retroactive payment for the years zakat was not distributed.

A recent policy change announced an increase in zakat grants. For some time, the grant had been Rs. 900 a quarter or Rs. 300 per month. Beginning with the allocation at the end of 1999, the grants will be 1500 Rs. a recipient for three months.

On March 9, 1999, the Supreme Court of Pakistan decided that even Hanafi Muslims could be exempted from zakat collection if they filed a form with their bank that said that their faith did not require them to pay zakat. In the case of the *Government of Pakistan, Finance Division et al. vs. Farzana Asar,* the court found that accepting the declaration of the Shias, but not accepting the declaration of a Hanafi Muslim, was "violative of the inalienable fundamental rights of being treated in accordance with the law and equality before the law guaranteed under Articles 4 and 25 of the Constitution." Henceforth, banks will have to accept the declaration of any Pakistani Muslim that he or she believes that government collection of zakat would violate his or her belief in Islam. This ruling has the potential to undermine Pakistan's entire zakat system, since Sunni Muslims can now decide they do not wish to pay zakat to the government. Indications from the zakat collections in December 1999 suggest that zakat collections are down compared to previous collections.

Previous Evaluation of Pakistan's Zakat System

Only a few people have written previously attempting to evaluate the actual impact of Pakistan's system. In 1985, Clark wrote her doctoral dissertation on Pakistan's zakat as a social welfare system. In 1983-84 she found that the system was not financially adequate to provide for people's needs, but that the system helped recipients to eat better and to have a few modest comforts for their lives, such as letter writing, tea, warm second-hand clothes for winter, or cooking oil. She also found that while the system helped many desperately poor people, there was nowhere near enough money to help all those who needed help. Rehabilitation efforts were minimal and mostly focused on buying sewing machines for women and tools for men. There was very minimal support for health care or dowries. Clark also found that while many people were skeptical of President Zia's motives for initiating zakat, most people supported the concept of zakat and the payment of zakat to the very poor, especially the elderly.

In 1990, Faiz Mohammad (1990) conducted a survey on zakat. He found that only two percent of recipients felt the amounts received were adequate. Only 16 percent of those who received rehabilitation grants believed them to be adequate. Following up on this evaluation, the Central Zakat Administration did its own evaluation of the zakat system (Government of Pakistan, 1991). While the Central Zakat Administration considers this report secret, Shirazi (1996) reported in his own book that the management study found extensive corruption in the form of payments to relatives, partial payments to recipients, zakat payments diverted to politics, and other irregularities. The report also found that persons who owed zakat were moving their assets just before Ramadan to avoid payment of zakat.

Shirazi's own appraisal of zakat provides another broad view of Pakistan's zakat up to 1994. Using secondary data from the economic census and studies of caloric intake, he concluded that zakat had increased the caloric intake of Pakistan's lowest income group and decreased the poverty gap between two to three percent. Unfortunately, his data did not include the very poorest Pakistanis who would be the most likely targets for zakat. Also, he did not perform any analysis by age groups.

Shirazi also found that the Government of Pakistan did not disburse all of the money it collected every year, but built up an account over time. This account was invested in Islamic banks. Still, it was invested, and the government received a return on it, contrary to Islamic law. By 1994, the government had accrued a balance of about Rs. 10 billion that had not gone to zakat recipients.

In 1997, Abdullah, head of the Rural Development Academy in Peshawar, presented a paper at a development conference in Beijing in which he claimed that zakat had helped to eliminate poverty in Pakistan. His basic thesis was that Islamic institutions are the solution to eliminating poverty in developing nations. He presented Pakistan's zakat as a system that has raised the living standard of Pakistanis. He presented data allegedly from the Ministry of Religious Affairs from 1990 through 1996 about nationwide zakat collections and disbursements by province, but he made no mention that at the time he presented his paper, zakat had not been distributed in N.W.F.P., his own province, for two years (Abdullah, 1997).

Evaluation of the Impact of Zakat at This Time

In 1999 and 2000, the author returned to Pakistan to study what changes had occurred in the national zakat and ushr system since 1984 and to study zakat as a resource for the elderly poor. Of particular interest was the opportunity to see what impact zakat had had within the intervening years both in terms of the original stated goals, and in terms of unforeseen impacts in any other areas.

Goal 1: Zakat Would Provide Financial Assistance to Those in Need and Who Could Not Work

Two important concepts in evaluating this goal are "adequacy" and "efficiency." "Adequacy" is the degree to which the benefits received are sufficient to provide for the recipient's needs. "Efficiency" is the degree to which the actual distribution of income coincides with the desired redistribution, or the degree to which the system meets the needs of all who are technically eligible, while excluding those not eligible (Marmor, 1971).

In terms of adequacy, Pakistan's zakat system has never been adequate to meet the subsistence needs of those who receive it. The modal grant of Rs.100 per month in 1984 (then equal to $3) was considered inadequate by the overwhelming majority of those connected with the system, and by all recipients. Today's modal grant of Rs. 300 per month (now $6) is still inadequate. Even with the increase to Rs. 500 ($10) per month, an income of Rs. 6000 per year ($120) is far below what one would need to meet basic needs in Pakistan.

In 1994, Pakistan's poverty line, defined as the minimum income needed per capita to meet basic needs, was Rs. 384 per month, with Rs. 450 in urban areas and Rs. 343 in rural areas (Mahbub ul-Haq Center for International Development, 1999). At that time the modal monthly grant was Rs. 200. Unfortunately, more recent household figures to determine what is the poverty line for 1999 do not exist, but with the inflation of recent years, the poverty line is now probably at least Rs. 800 to 1000.

According to the recent poverty study by the Mahbub ul-Haq Centre for Human Development (1999), 28.6 percent of Pakistan's people lived below the poverty line in 1986/87, while 35.7 percent lived below the poverty line in 1993/94. Throughout this period poverty indicators fluctuated from year to year in direct proportion to the economy. While the Centre notes that the poor have occasionally been selectively targeted by different government programs, "more often they have been the lucky recipients of high growth fallout rather than the intended recipients of conscious state policy" (p. 3). The report also noted that throughout Pakistan, "poverty has a predominantly female face" (p. 6). Female-headed households are consistently poorer than male-headed households. This is consistent with the pattern of zakat recipients who, except for the students who receive zakat, are predominantly female. Unfortunately, the study does not identify the proportion of elderly who are poor.

Adequacy, however, is a relative concept. While the zakat grant may not be adequate to meet basic needs, it is much better than absolutely no cash income at all. What the zakat amount does do is to give the recipient a few choices about her life. Most people in Pakistan will give a poor old man or old widow a piece of bread if asked, but the money from zakat means that a person can also buy some fruit and vegetables, some lentils or milk. It means that a person has the possibility to buy needed medicine. It means that the recipient can buy some second-hand clothes, or shoes, or a coat for winter.

The effect on families is fairly subtle. Many elderly receiving zakat live alone, which is itself unusual in Pakistan. Zakat enables them to reestablish some communication with family members who have moved to the city or another village. This helps to reduce the loneliness and isolation that many of them report. About half the elderly recipients live with a distant relative or non-relative who is also very poor. The addition of even Rs. 300 a month to the family's joint income helps the household as a whole and tends to increase the status of the zakat recipient within the household, particularly widows. Many report more respect once they began receiving zakat.

On the other hand, zakat is not adequate in that it is neither predictable nor reliable. Theoretically, once someone is named a zakat recipient, she should be able to count on zakat payments quarterly until she dies or her situation changes. This is not the case. Zakat is not disbursed to the provinces, or districts, or LZCs on a regular basis. Often long periods of time lapse from one disbursement to the next.

The most egregious instance of inadequate grants was the three-year suspension of zakat payments for most of Pakistan. During this time zakat recipients who had previously been determined to be desperately poor received no income from zakat. It is not known if any people died of starvation or exposure because of this, or how many. When Justice Mirza, Chairman of the Central Zakat Council, was asked about this, he said that people probably did die, but that the government was not legally liable for people who died as a result of a change of policy (1999). Moreover, zakat is not an entitlement, but a gift. Recipients cannot plan for the future, because they don't know if they will continue to receive zakat in the future or not. Then, too, zakat distribution is based on the committee's decision of who gets it, not necessarily who is neediest.

Adequacy is further reduced by the imposition of bank fees on the recipients. Most banks require that recipients keep a minimum of Rs. 500 in their accounts, although for some banks the minimum amount is Rs. 1000. This keeps money that is supposed to belong to the recipient tied up in the bank and not available for use. It means that the real first payment to the zakat recipients after going without any payment for three years was Rs. 400 for the quarter instead of Rs. 900.

One of the major limitations of the system is that all recipients receive the same amount, no matter where they live in Pakistan or how many people the grant must support. Thus, a widow alone receives Rs. 500. If an old man cannot work to support himself and his wife, he receives Rs. 500 for both of them. A young widow with five small children also receives Rs. 500. Moreover, there is no differentiation in rates between different temperature regions of Pakistan. The same amount goes to recipients in tropical areas of Pakistan, where it is possible to grow food all year long and where it is never cold as to areas such as Chital in the Himalayas, where it is brutally cold in the winter, requiring warm clothes, fuel, and more food calories to stay warm.

In terms of efficiency, Marmor (1971) differentiates two types of efficiency. Vertical efficiency is the extent to which the program benefits those who are not targeted, that is, unintended beneficiaries. Horizontal efficiency is the extent to which the program reaches intended beneficiaries, i.e., the groups specified in zakat's legal mandate.

To begin with horizontal efficiency, Pakistan's zakat program is targeted at the very poorest of widows, orphans and the handicapped and disabled. Almost all of the people who actually receive zakat are eligible for it. The problem is that there are far more people eligible than there are funds to disburse. As mentioned above, about 34% of Pakistan's population lived below the poverty line in 1994.

Because the question of who are the most deserving needy persons in the village is a judgment call, many factors influence who receives zakat in addition to financial need. Most of the LZCs visited and surveyed report that they receive from two to three times more requests for assistance than they can provide. Some requests are determined to be inappropriate, but many are determined to be needy, just not as deserving, for whatever reason, as someone else. Some of the factors committees report using in determining deservedness are: (1) Whether or not the person is physically or socially capable of supporting him or herself; (2) Whether or not the person is a "good Muslim," usually defined as much by day to day moral behavior as much or more than religious observance *per se*; (3) What the person has contributed to others during his lifetime; (4) In the case of orphans, the child's potential gifts which could be useful for the community if given economic support; (5) Whether or not the potential recipient has male relatives who should be supporting them, especially local male relatives.

Moreover, most districts impose a limit of ten grantees per quarter per LZC, whether the LZC area is rich or poor. In very poor areas, there may be many more than 10 people who are needy and eligible. Also, the program puts needy seniors in competition with the handicapped and young widows with children as well as students. While most LZCs report giving priority to impoverished older widows, so that over half of the zakat recipients fall into this group, other LZCs believe that the money should go to support young fatherless families or to education, so there is no guarantee that a widow with no income at all will receive zakat.

Vertical efficiency has to do with unintended beneficiaries. Many groups of people benefit from zakat who are not the law's intended targets. These include:

1. The Government of Pakistan—Pakistan's government has for some years been under tremendous pressure from the World Bank and donor agencies to improve its financial practices and its liquid reserves. It would appear that from 1995 until the present, the Government of Pakistan used zakat money to help solve its liquidity crisis and to help pay for other priorities. This is also absolutely illegal under Pakistani law and immoral under Islamic law, but neither of these factors seems to have been an impediment. While it was the Finance Ministry who originally appropriated the zakat money into the consolidated fund, officials at the Ministry for Re-

ligious Affairs have gone along with this arrangement for several years. The amount of zakat funds used this way was estimated to be Rs. 14 billion (U.S. $70 million) in addition to the Rs. 10 billion that had accrued prior to 1994.

Although this policy began with the second government of Benazir Bhutto in 1995, the government of Nawaz Sharif continued it. The Sharif government reconstituted the local zakat committees and began to disburse zakat again, but they and the present government have continued to use some of the zakat money collected to help with liquidity.

2. Banks–Banks benefit in two ways that were not originally intended. First, banks use the float from zakat funds deposited with them until the recipients can withdraw their money. A single quarter's zakat deposits would be about Rs. 200 million. It is in the bank's financial interest to make this process as difficult as possible, since the longer the money stays in the accounts, the more money the bank can use as float. In addition, the banks receive the Rs. 500 per recipient fee for opening an account. If one calculates Rs. 500 per person times 400,000 recipients, it comes to another Rs. 200 million that the banks have received as profit. Note that the Rs. 500 collected for administrative purposes is not float. It is profit that goes directly to the bank in addition to float.

3. Members of LZC committees who take a "surcharge for administrative costs"–This is illegal under Pakistan's law, and immoral in Islamic law, but some committees themselves report that they do this. What is heartening are the large number of committees who really do work hard for no pay at all and who even pay money out of their own pocket for needy persons when there is no zakat money available.

4. Some relatives and friends or political supporters of LZC members–Some areas report that LZCs favor their own poor relatives over other deserving persons. It is not completely clear whether the relatives are technically eligible or not, but there is clear community sentiment that the relatives are not the most needy. This sort of favoritism appears to have increased since the appointment of LZC chairs on the basis of politics.

5. Political parties in power–These parties now dole out chairmanships of LZCs like any other political patronage. In Pakistan, political patronage often leads to graft and corruption, since the expectation exists that appointed positions will result in personal profit.

6. Thieves–As with any large amount of money, some people simply steal it. One person responsible for the federal administration of zakat absconded to London with a billion rupees of zakat money.

Goal 2: The Zakat System Would Provide Economic Rehabilitation for Those Who Could Work

Western welfare systems worry about the disincentives to work that a welfare system brings. Most recipients of zakat are not regarded locally as good candidates for work in the first place, especially older widows or very young children. A few, especially younger widows and the handicapped, both men and women, are able to receive training through zakat "rehabilitation grants." When zakat first began, these were common. LZCs could decide for themselves who would receive such a grant, usually about Rs. 5000 (U.S. $100, although in the 1980s, Rs. 5000 was more like $300). Since a majority of the LZCs surveyed in 1984 reported at least one rehabilitation grant throughout the previous year, these grants were relatively extensive.

Now these grants are decided at the DZC level, on the recommendation of the LZC. Only four percent of the funds disbursed to the DZC is spent on rehabilitation. Almost all of this money goes to handicapped men and young widows, or orphaned girls. Usually the grant consists of training and the minimal amount required for equipment, materials, and supplies to start up a very small business. Older men and women rarely receive a rehabilitation grant. For the vulnerable elderly receiving zakat, however, there is little expectation that they would be working if they did not receive zakat or that they should work.

Goal 3: Zakat Would Eliminate Beggary

This goal makes the assumption that beggary is related directly to poverty, a somewhat naïve assumption. While many people in Pakistan may be driven to beggary initially because of desperate poverty, except for some beggars in small villages, there is little free-lance beggary in Pakistan. Most beggars are organized into groups, sometimes families. These organized groups provide protection for the beggars and co-ordinate who will be allowed to beg at which spot. The groups also pay bribes to police, if necessary, to allow them to continue to beg in a particular place. The beggars themselves receive some portion of what they collect, with the remainder going to the organization. Usually beggars in these organized groups are at least guaranteed some food and shelter, although the beggars themselves are at the mercy of the group leaders.

Once in these beggary groups, there is little opportunity to leave. If they could find a job, they would have. If their families would have helped them, they would not have had to turn to beggary, and once they become beggars, their families want nothing to do with them. Beggars live in the marginal world of social outcasts. Children of beggars often are initiated into the begging system at an early age. Because of their highly stigmatized social status, beggars tend to marry each other and beget another generation of beggars.

Fluctuations in the appearance of beggars on the street have to do with a number of factors in addition to the economy. Perhaps the largest factor is the policy of the government of the moment in relation to beggars. If the policy is "no beggars" and the police enforce that policy, the number of beggars on the street decreases markedly. Meanwhile, the beggar organizations can turn to other socially marginal ways to make money until the enforcement drive slackens or a new government comes in with new priorities.

Thus, beggary was seen much less under President Zia ul-Haq than currently because of a stronger enforcement of anti-beggary laws rather than because of zakat. What the presence of zakat did do was to allow the police to have public support for stricter enforcement of anti-beggary laws because people believed that zakat existed to take care of the people who were begging.

What zakat may do is to prevent some people from entering into beggary, although there have been no thorough studies of what causes people to turn to beggary. Most of the people who collect zakat consider themselves "respectable." While they feel comfortable asking relatives and neighbors for help, which is usually the whole population of a small village, many would, literally, die before they would join the world of the highly stigmatized organized beggars. A study undertaken by the National Council of Social Welfare in 1999 found that beggars did not want to answer questions because they were afraid. Data that was collected was highly suspect, and the study fizzled out (Zaman, 1999).

Goal 4: Zakat Would Redistribute the Wealth in the Society

Political idealists advocating for zakat see it as a vehicle to redistribute wealth in the society so that no one is poor. They see the Islamic injunction of giving zakat to those who cannot work as a Godly commandment as well as a way of circulating money in the society.

Pakistan's zakat has redistributed wealth from the rich to the poor, but only in the most modest sense. The amount of money collected by the zakat system represents a very small portion of the assets of the society. While the elderly have benefited from this redistribution more than any other group, even the money redistributed to them has been very modest.

For most of Pakistan's existence, it has experienced a growth rate of about six percent a year. This was more than enough to increase the standard of living of everyone in the society. Instead, while the rich in Pakistan have become much richer, the poor have remained poor and increased in number, with 34 percent living below the basic needs poverty line in 1994. The wealth, which has been developed in Pakistan over this time, has not gone to aid the poor or to build a public infrastructure or public services that would benefit the poor. Rather, most of Pakistan's increasing wealth has gone to already rich individuals (Mahbub ul-Haq Centre, 1999). Corruption at all levels of government has resulted in redistributing income from economic growth to those in positions of power.

Pakistan's early experiences with zakat, however, do demonstrate that zakat has the potential to redistribute wealth in the society.

Goal 5: The Zakat System Would Eliminate Poverty

Pakistan's zakat system has not eliminated poverty. Some Islamic theorists may argue that this is because Pakistan did not institute zakat on a large enough base of assets to insure sufficient funds to make a major dent in poverty (K. Ahmad, 1980; Siddiqi, 1983). While there is some truth to this argument, it ignores the residual nature of poverty.

For the most part, poverty in any society is a function of opportunities available to people as much as money. Even though Pakistan has had an excellent growth rate for most of its existence, the failure to provide educational, health and job opportunities to millions of its citizens has resulted in persistent poverty (Mahbub ul-Haq Centre, 1999). No amount of zakat as a subsistence payment can make up for a lack of education or the denial of medical treatment that would enable a person to be truly self-sufficient.

While Shirazi (1996) found that zakat helped to narrow the poverty gap slightly, about 2.9 percent in the years he studied, he documented that, in fact, zakat had not eliminated poverty. With 34 percent of its people living below the poverty line, there is no way that Pakistan can claim that anything has eliminated poverty. While zakat has clearly not eliminated poverty in Pakistan, it was unrealistic to expect it to do so. At best, zakat, like other welfare systems, was set up to alleviate poverty, not to prevent it.

Goal 6: The Government Would Be More Conscientious About Running a Program Based on Important Islamic Beliefs

Of all the goals and expectations set for Pakistan's zakat system, this has been the greatest failure. In the beginning, there was the inherent belief that an Islamic system that focused on goals of social justice would be exempt from greed, politics, and corruption. This proved to be a naïve expectation. While initially there may have been some isolated instances of misappropriation of funds, most people involved in the zakat system were conscientious about managing the system to the best of their ability. Over time, however, this conscientiousness eroded until the misappropriation of zakat funds became part of the national government's policy.

When zakat first began, it was one of the few Islamization measures that had widespread support, because people believed that it had some hope of helping the very poorest people. Even at the beginning, there was fear of corruption, but the CZA made many efforts to be publicly accountable, and to follow up on stories of corruption. Zakat funds were maintained in a separate account, used only for zakat. Even funds for the administration of zakat, technically allowable under Islamic law, were provided out of the consolidated fund rather than zakat funds (Clark, 1985).

In the intervening years, public support for the zakat system has decreased. Few people begrudge zakat to the very poor, but more and more people do not trust the government to deliver zakat money. The withholding of zakat for three years shows these fears to be well founded. Most people still are not aware that the federal government withheld zakat for three years. When this knowledge becomes widespread, public support for zakat likely will decrease even further.

It is hard to imagine how cynical one would have to be to be an official in the Ministry for Religious Affairs, responsible for supporting Islamic institutions, and go along with withholding zakat from widows and orphans. Of all the people in Pakistan, these are the people most likely to be able to cite the Chapters and verses of the Quran that explicitly forbid this. At the same time, the evidence suggests that these officials went along with the government's policies to withhold zakat from poor people, and that they are continuing to withhold large amounts of what is collected. There is no evidence to suggest one way or another whether any of them profited financially from this themselves, although they profited personally in the sense that they all kept their jobs.

To summarize this analysis, Pakistan's national zakat system has enormous potential to help vulnerable poor older Pakistanis, but that potential is being undermined through a variety of factors including insufficient funding, a cumbersome administrative process, and corruption. At the present time, zakat has had some positive impact to help Pakistan's poorest Muslim citizens to survive and to lead at least marginally better lives, but its potential to continue to do so is decreasing with the decrease in public support.

CONCLUSION

Pakistan's national zakat system has shown that such a system can be used to redistribute money for subsistence for older persons. Pakistan has demonstrated that a relatively poor country can provide a simple safety net for the most vulnerable of the elderly poor.

Pakistan's zakat system began by espousing the highest of ideals based on traditional Islamic law. Early implementation showed that it had the potential to help hundreds of thousands of very poor and vulnerable Pakistanis. It demonstrated that it had the capacity to attract hundreds of thousands of sincere Muslims to participate in the administration of the system on a voluntary basis.

Administratively, Pakistan has shown great creativity in using some modern concepts and techniques to implement the system. Pakistan simplified zakat collection enormously by using existing banking structures and computers to collect the zakat rather than setting up a separate collection structure. Pakistan also showed great creativity in using local committees of volunteers rather than paid staff, thus reducing overhead costs.

In 2000, Pakistan's national zakat system had over 40,000 local zakat committees, each of which provided some subsistence to at least 10 persons. The majority of those persons, at least 200,000 people, were vulnerable elderly. This means that 3% of Pakistan's elderly received some income from this system. For almost all of them, that money was the only cash income that they received to help survive.

While zakat did not set out to be a financial safety net for elderly persons, the practical impact of the system is that it is the closest thing to such a safety net that Pakistan has for its older citizens. Pakistan has demonstrated that even a very poor country can begin to use existing indigenous structures and concepts to create a workable system that helps the elderly to survive.

Pakistan's zakat system has serious flaws. Much would need to be done to make zakat the vehicle for major redistribution of wealth in the society, or even to make it a reliable source for subsistence, especially to the elderly poor. With all its flaws, however, the zakat system does manage to provide essential help to about 3% of Pakistan's elderly. In this limited sense, it does serve as a system to redistribute wealth to the elderly poor.

Other countries considering a national zakat system could replicate some of the positive aspects of Pakistan's zakat, while avoiding the pitfalls that Pakistan has experienced. By reviewing both positive and negative aspects of Pakistan's experience, policymakers in other Muslim countries may be able to make a more informed decision about the use of a national zakat system in redistributing wealth to elderly poor persons in their countries.

REFERENCES

Abdullah. (1997). *Pakistan's poverty lessons and integrative remedies.* Monograph presented at Regional Expert Group Meeting at Beijing, China, March 26, 1997.

Afzul, M. (1999). *The situation of elderly people in Pakistan.* New York: United Nations.

Afzal ur-Rahman. (1974). *Economic doctrines of Islam.* Lahore: Islamic Publications.

Aghnides, N. (1981). *An introduction to Mohammedan Law.* Lahore: Sang-e-Meel Publications.

Al-Qardawi, A.Y. (1981). *Economic security in Islam.* Translated by M.I. Siddiqi. Lahore: Kazi Publications.

Belokrenitsky, V. (1984). Rural-urban migration and the urban poor in Pakistan. *Journal of South Asian and Middle Eastern Studies*, VIII:1:35-46.

Clark, G. (1985). *Pakistan's zakat: An Islamic public welfare system in a developing country.* Unpublished thesis, University of Maryland School of Social Work and Community Planning. 1985.

Clark, G. and H. Zaman. (2000). *Preliminary report on the findings of the Pakistan Aging Survey.* Islamabad: National Council of Social Welfare.

Crane, R.D. (1981). *Islamic commercial law and contemporary economics.* Washington, D.C.: Department of State.

Dar, R.H. (1996). *Status of the aged in modernising society.* Master's thesis. Sociology Department of the University of the Punjab. Unpublished.

Faiz, M. (1990). *Evaluation of Nizam-e-Zakat and Ushr in Pakistan.* Islamabad: International Islamic University.

Government of Pakistan, Central Zakat Administration. (1991). *Zakat and Ushr.* Islamabad: Government of Pakistan.

Government of Pakistan, *Finance Division vs. Fazana Asar,* Decision of the Supreme Court of Pakistan, March 9, 1999.

Government of Pakistan. (1980). *Report of the Committee on Islamization.* Islamabad: Institute of Development Economics.

Government of Pakistan Population Census Organization, Statistics Division (1999). *Advance tabulation on sex, age group, marital status, and educational attainment.* Islamabad: Government of Pakistan.

Government of Pakistan (1980). *Zakat and Ushr Ordinance of 1980.* Islamabad: Government of Pakistan.

Haddad, Y. (1982). The Islamic Alternative. In *The Link*, 15: 4. (September/October).

Imtiazi, I.A. Personal interview in Lahore, August 1999.

Khan, A.K. (Ed.). (1983). *Manual of Zakat and Ushr Laws.* Lahore: C.C.L. Publications.

Khan, D. (1981). Planning for the poor in Pakistan: Rhetoric and reality. In R.P. Misra (Ed.), *Humanizing development.* Singapore: Maruzan Asia.

Mahbub ul-Haq Centre for Human Development. (1999). *Profile of poverty in Pakistan.* Islamabad: United Nations Development Program.

Mannon, M.A. (1980). *Islamic economics: Theory and practice.* Lahore: Sh. Muhammad Ashraf.

Marmor, T. (1971). On comparing income maintenance policy alternatives. *Political Science Review*, 65: 971: 83-96.

Maududi, S.A. (1978). *First principles of the Islamic state.* Lahore: Islamic Publications.

Mirza, Mr. Justice Munawar. Interview. Islamabad, April 1999.

Qureshi, A.H., Administrator Zakat, Person Interview in Islamabad, March, 1999.

Qureshi, A.I. (1979). *The economic and social system of Islam.* Lahore: Islamic Book Service.

Sabzwari, M.A. (1979). *A study of Zakat and Ushr with special reference to Pakistan.* Karachi: Industries Printing Press.

Shirazi, N.S. (1996). *System of Zakat in Pakistan.* Islamabad: International Institute of Islamic Economics.

Siddiqui, M.A.S. (1983). *Early development of Zakat Law and Ijtahad.* Karachi: Islamic Research Academy.

Tanzil-ur-Rahman. (1981). *Introduction of Zakat system in Pakistan.* Islamabad: Council of Islamic Ideology.

U.S. Department of Commerce, Bureau of the Census. (1996). *Global aging into the 21st century.* Washington, D.C.: GPO.

Zaman, H. (1999). *A study of beggary in Islamabad* (a research report). Islamabad: National Council of Social Welfare.

Zia ul-Haq. (1980). Introduction of Zakat in Pakistan. (English translation of a speech in Urdu at the Jamia Masjid). Islamabad, June 20, 1980.

PART II:
RELIGION, SPIRITUALITY, AND AGING

In this section, we explore how religion and spirituality influence individuals, families, organizations, and governments. More and more, we have become aware of the importance of belief systems, values, and culture in understanding and dealing with the challenges brought about by advancing age. The elderly employ belief systems and tradition to comprehend the meaning of life as they seek answers to the questions of mortality and the afterlife. We know from much research that individuals with a strong value system are better equipped to deal with these questions than persons without a strong ideological base. Too, we are cognizant of how values and oftentimes religion itself mold and design organizational and governmental policies and programs for the elderly, as we have seen in the case of Pakistan's Zakat system. Today, in any discussion of aging, it is most important to consider the influence and effects of religion, spirituality, and other belief systems upon individuals, families, programs, and policies.

We have in this section a number of examples of the integration of religion and spirituality with aging concerns. Dr. Sassy Sasson of The Jewish Home and Hospital presents the results of his study of religiosity, adjustment, and satisfaction of a select group of nursing home residents. He found that elders with higher levels of religiosity showed greater levels of adjustment and satisfaction to their situations in the nursing home. Related to this finding, he opines, is the continuance of previous religious practices, roles, and behaviors. Dr. Sasson uses these findings to draw programmatic implications for long-term residents of nursing homes.

We also have a similar study of African American and Latino groups by Elizabeth Bertera and Barbara Bailey-Etta, Assistant Professors at the Catholic University of America. Using samples drawn from the National Health and Nutrition Examination Survey (NHANES III), they investigate how these racial and ethnic groups differ in social participation activities, degree of physical dysfunction, and church and/or club attendance. They recommend a wide range of social work interventions designed to improve the quality of life for older Americans, especially African Americans and Latinos.

Another paper introduces logotherapy and concepts developed by Victor Frankl as tools in defining the meaning of life by older persons. David Guttmann, Professor Emeritus at Haifa University, Israel, elaborates on Frankl's notions of guilt, suffering, and death as unavoidable factors in life that lead to understanding and meaning. Further, the spirituality of old age is explored. In a similar vein, Gerson David, Professor at the University of Houston, indicates that in today's world, a discussion of aging must include a discussion of religion and spirituality. Introducing a spiritual model based on Hinduism, he posits that the meaning of life is gained from religion and spirituality. Dr. David concludes with suggestions for how social workers and other caregivers might understand and discuss religion, spirituality, and the meaning of life with the elderly.

In our final article, JoAnn Burke of St. Mary's College, Notre Dame, Indiana writes of the challenges of a group of Catholic nuns who unexpectedly and without preparation were called home to care for an elderly parent. Dr. Burke utilizes role theory to examine the conditions under which the demands of parental care arose, the types of care offered, and the conflict between their religious and caregiving roles. She concludes by offering suggestions that address this reality.

In conclusion, we have offered this volume entitled *Issues in Global Aging* as a resource for students, social work practitioners and caretakers of the elderly, agency administrators, policy-makers, and researchers in the field of gerontology. It is our hope that it may assist them in a better understanding of global concerns that we all face in meeting the needs of the elderly today. Daniel Thursz advised us to empower the elderly as they seek access to work, income, health care, and shelter. He would agree with the authors in this volume that in crafting policies to address the needs of the elderly throughout the world, we must keep in mind the importance of peace and human rights. Also I am sure that he would concur that tradition, culture, values, religion, and spirituality are crucial variables in addressing and resolving these issues and concerns.

Religiosity
as a Factor Affecting Adjustment
of Minority Elderly to a Nursing Home

Sassy Sasson

SUMMARY. This study examines the association between religiosity, adjustment and satisfaction of nursing home residents in one long term care facility. A sample of convenience was used to conduct face-to-face interviews of 71 Jewish and 21 African American alert residents age 65 and older. Various scales were utilized to measure resident adjustment and satisfaction, religious identity and level of involvement in religious activities. Additional information was compiled that provided a profile of the physical, mental and social functions of each resident. The findings revealed that residents who exhibit higher levels of religiosity were likely to show higher levels of adjustment and satisfaction with nursing home living. However, the results lost their significance after controlling for a variety of other characteristics. The results suggest that the continuation of previous religious roles, activities and behavior of nursing home residents may prompt increased satisfaction and a more successful ad-

Sassy Sasson, DSW, CSW, is affiliated with The Jewish Home and Hospital, 100 West Kingsbridge Road, Bronx, NY 10468.

The author gratefully acknowledges the contributions of Arlene Nelson-Sasson, CSW, Dr. Eileen Chichin, Dr. Norman Linzer, Dr. David Schnall and Dr. James Schmeidler. An earlier version of this paper was presented at the 53rd Annual Scientific Meeting of the Gerontological Society of America, November 2000, Washington, DC.

[Haworth co-indexing entry note]: "Religiosity as a Factor Affecting Adjustment of Minority Elderly to a Nursing Home." Sasson, Sassy. Co-published simultaneously in *Social Thought* (The Haworth Press, Inc.) Vol. 20, No. 3/4, 2001, pp. 79-96; and: *Issues in Global Aging* (ed: Frederick L. Ahearn, Jr.) The Haworth Press, Inc., 2001, pp. 79-96. Single or multiple copies of this article are available for a fee from The Haworth Document Delivery Service [1-800-HAWORTH, 9:00 a.m. - 5:00 p.m. (EST). E-mail address: getinfo@haworthpressinc.com].

justment to the long term care setting. The implications of these findings for practice, program development and future research will be discussed. *[Article copies available for a fee from The Haworth Document Delivery Service: 1-800-HAWORTH. E-mail address: <getinfo@haworthpressinc.com> Website: <http://www.HaworthPress.com> © 2001 by The Haworth Press, Inc. All rights reserved.]*

KEYWORDS. Religiosity, adjustment, satisfaction, coping, well-being

INTRODUCTION

Despite the consistent growth of knowledge and information in the area of religion and aging, research efforts have been minimal in exploring the impact of religiosity upon the adjustment of nursing home residents stemming from diverse ethnic groups (Cohen, Hyland & Magal, 1998). Within the institutional setting, personal belief systems and practices often become secondary to professionals in their daily care of residents. Elderly individuals whose ethnic identity is an integral part of their existence may feel isolated in their particular customs and habits. This may ultimately affect their level of adjustment to the environment.

Various attempts have been made to examine the effects of religion upon the physical and mental health of older adults. Attendance at religious services was positively correlated with the variables of health, health status and functional capacity (Mull, Cox & Sullivan, 1987). Additionally, greater intrinsic religiosity independently predicted a shorter time to remission of depression in medically ill older patients (Koenig, George & Peterson, 1998). Moreover, adults who partake in private prayer evidence a significant decrease in symptoms of depression and general distress one year after undergoing coronary bypass surgery (Ai, Dunkle, Peterson & Bolling, 1998). Religious coping was also found to be a common behavior among older medical inpatients and was inversely related to depression among elderly men (Koenig, Cohen, Blazer, Pieper, Meador, Shelp, Goli & DiPasquale, 1992).

Two distinct ethnic groups were chosen to examine the potency of religiosity in determining the adjustment and satisfaction of ethnically and racially different older adults to nursing home living. This article discusses the association between religiosity and adjustment among African American and Jewish nursing home residents and the differences between these groups in one long term care facility. The results of the study may be useful for the development of formal and informal mechanisms which will enhance the adjustment and satisfaction of residents in the nursing home milieu, while promoting their spiritual, physical and emotional well-being.

Religion and Adjustment to the Nursing Home

Relocation to a nursing home is a significant life change for any older adult. Institutional living requires changes in lifestyle, social network, customs and food, and is accompanied by the loss of privacy and independence. Departure from a nurturing and familiar environment diminishes the individual's sense of autonomy, and often impacts upon his/her self-esteem (Butler, 1985). This may activate feelings of anger, abandonment, frustration, isolation, hopelessness and despair, often leading to a depressed mood (Ames, 1991). At this crucial time, involvement in religious activities may help ease the transition and can help older adults adapt to this major change in later life.

Adjustment to a long term care facility can be a difficult process for the older adult. In addition to the loss of a similar community and its customs, elders must now adhere to the nursing home rules, norms, culture and practices. A myriad of factors determine the type of adjustment that one may experience. The level of acclimation to nursing home living may be affected by the resident's social class (Redfoot, 1987), self-efficacy and locus of control (Johnson, Stone, Altmaier & Berdahl, 1998), gender (Joiner & Freudiger, 1993), family support (Shanas, 1979), and a positive attitude towards nursing home care (Mui & Burnette, 1994). Furthermore, adjustment difficulties can be attributed to the older adult's capacity for interpersonal relationships, level of social isolation, marital status, level of independence, attitude toward admission and psychiatric history (Rodstein, Savitsky & Starkman, 1976).

Religion is often a factor that positively affects the older person's adjustment to later life (Koenig, Smiley & Gonzales, 1988). It is a central facet of life for an older person as it serves as a source of strength, comfort and inspiration during difficult times. In fact, prayer is utilized more frequently among older adults than in other age groups (Levin & Taylor, 1997). Empirical studies reveal a significant association between participation in religious activities and morale, happiness, usefulness and quality of life (Blazer & Palmore, 1976; Ellison & Gay, 1990).

The transition to a nursing home environment can be conceived as a stressful life event for the older adult. Ellison (1994) provides a theoretical construct which links religious factors with the components of the life stress paradigm. He argues that aspects of religious involvement may elicit several positive manifestations and reduce the risk for depression and other psychiatric disorders. The therapeutic results of religious involvement are construed as: (1) the reduction of the risk of exposure to certain stressors; (2) the provision of cognitive and institutional frameworks that reduce the rate of certain stressors to the older individual; (3) the increase of values and awareness of various social resources; (4) the enhancement of valuable psychological resources, particularly positive self-perceptions.

Religiosity is an aspect of life that may enhance the experiences and overall quality of life of older persons. Moberg (1970) suggests two orientations to religion. An institutional orientation applies to group related behaviors such as types of religious rituals, e.g., attendance at church/synagogue. A personal orientation reflects individual beliefs, values and attitudes. The ability to derive satisfaction and meaning from a religious role may impact upon the resident's contentment with nursing home living and heighten his/her ability to adapt to the multiple changes that arise. Within the nursing home milieu, a resident can maintain a religious role by reading Holy Scriptures, praying privately, or attending religious services. This involvement can also facilitate the formation of relationships with members of their own group, which may produce emotional and instrumental support. In fact, participation in religious activities were significantly associated with an increase in morale, social support and subjective coping (Koenig, Kvale & Ferrel, 1988).

Religion Among the African American and Jewish Elderly

The empirical literature confirms the centrality of religious participation in the personal lives of many black Americans. Jacobson, Heaton and Dennis (1990) concluded that black elders are more likely to pray privately and to attend religious services more frequently than their white counterparts. Moreover, black older adults were clearly more religious than their white peers. Social class was positively associated with religiosity among the black subjects, but found insignificant for the white elders. On the contrary, other studies demonstrated that socioeconomic status was not significantly related to life satisfaction among older black Americans (Ellison & Gay, 1990).

Research reveals that older African American adults tend to evidence higher levels of religiosity and perceived social support than their peers of different ethnic origins (Husaini, Blasi & Miller, 1999). In fact, for this group religion symbolizes an important source of social support and a mechanism for coping with stressful life events (Stolley & Koenig, 1997). Church attendance rates are particularly high among African Americans. Additionally, involvement in religious activities was most prominent among the older age groups (Chatters & Taylor, 1989). Participation in organizational religiosity among African Americans was deemed significantly related to life satisfaction (Levin, Chatters & Taylor, 1995).

Although extensive research has been conducted on the effect that religiosity elicits regarding the health and well-being of African American elderly individuals, similar efforts have been minimal with regard to the examination of the Jewish elderly on these issues. Empirical studies suggest that Jews are higher utilizers of health services than non-Jews (Larson, Donahue, Lyons, Benson, Patison, Worthington & Blazer, 1989; Schiller & Levin, 1988). It has been reported that involvement in prayers may have a therapeutic influence on elderly Jews, and was found to be non-threatening for the cognitively impaired elderly (Abramowitz, 1993).

METHODOLOGY

Participants

The research method selected for the study is the single point in time cross-sectional survey. Residents were interviewed after the initial two months of their stay at the nursing home facility. The two-month period of admission was selected in order to avoid the "first months syndrome" and the difficulties that generally accompany new admissions (Joiner & Freudiger, 1993; Sigman, 1986; Tobin, 1995). Other criteria for selection of subjects of the study included chronological age of 65 and above and a score of 20 or more points on the Mini-Mental Status Exam–MMSE (Folstein, Folstein & McHugh, 1975). Participants had to demonstrate a level of cognitive awareness in order to sign the informed consent form and to respond to the questions appropriately. The sample MMSE average score totalled $M = 24.73$, $SD = 3.4$ and a range of 20-30 points.

The sample of convenience consists of 71 Jewish and 21 African American residents of one long term care facility located in the New York metropolitan area. This skilled non-profit institution is non-sectarian, comprises 816 beds and provides a continuum of services to over 5,000 elderly and their families in both inpatient and outpatient settings. Despite the predominant representation of Jewish residents, the nursing home possesses an open door admission policy for all ethnic and racial groups.

Measures

The dependent variable, adjustment to nursing home living, is an objective scoring instrument that was used by the social workers in their evaluation of resident performance in the following areas: overall adjustment, grievances issued to staff, participation in activities and satisfaction with life at the facility. These criteria were selected from existing literature on adjustment (Amen, 1959; Dick & Friedsam, 1963; Joiner, 1989; Joiner & Freudiger, 1993). This researcher added the following indicators of adjustment: conflicts with roommates and/or other residents, cooperation with staff, compliance with treatment plan and level of verbal contact with other residents or staff.

The adjustment criteria were rated in five categories on an ordinal scale, ranging from never to very frequent. A reliability analysis was performed for the adjustment scale and a correlation matrix was calculated for all eight items. All items correlated positively with each other. During this process, reliability coefficients (Cronbach's alpha) were calculated for all the indicators of adjustment. Consequently, the overall score of the eight items was .86 and deemed as a relatively high reliability coefficient score.

The dependent variable, resident level of satisfaction with nursing home living, was assessed by utilizing the Nursing Home Resident Questionnaire (NHRQ) developed by Kane, Riegler, Bell, Potter and Koshland (1982). This 14-item scale was designed to measure resident satisfaction with issues directly affecting their life at the nursing home, rather than general life satisfaction. An additional question evaluates the extent to which each respondent enjoys nursing home living. The instrument asked respondents to indicate how much they agree or disagree with the statements on a three point ordinal scale. The authors tested the reliability coefficients of the scale. The combined score of all 14 items measured .88 in Cronbach's alpha (Kane et al., 1982).

The independent variable, involvement in religious activities, was classified in two areas. Personal religious activity implies reading the Bible or another holy book, praying privately and watching or listening to a religious program (Blazer & Palmore, 1976). Institutional group related activities include attending religious services, praying with a group or with a spiritual leader and going to church or synagogue (Koenig, Kvale & Ferrel, 1988). The respondents were asked to indicate the frequency of participation in religious activities on a five point ordinal scale ranging from never to very frequent. The participants were also requested to define their level of religiosity on an ordinal scale, comprised of three categories ranging from very religious to not religious at all (Markides, Levin & Ray, 1987). Reliability coefficients (Cronbach's alpha) were calculated for all the religious activities. The six activities revealed a composite score of alpha = .87, indicating a relatively high reliability coefficient.

Additional independent variables incorporated into the study were demographic values such as age, gender, education, religion, length of stay, marital status, and number of living children. Other functional variables represented the level of ability to perform Activities of Daily Living and the Mini-Mental Status Exam. This pertinent information was extracted from the medical chart of each participant. Subjects were then requested to describe their level of family involvement on a four point ordinal measure ranging from not involved to very involved, frequency of visits from family or friends and conversations with family members. Lastly, subjects were asked to indicate their desire to relocate to the nursing home on a four-point scale, ranging from not at all to very much.

Data Collection

The researcher met with each social worker to explain the purpose of the study and criteria for selection of subjects. Each unit social worker was requested to identify the residents who met the predetermined criteria for participation. The list of potential candidates was given to the researcher who subsequently, approached each resident to obtain their consent to participate in the study. The researcher also provided an explanation of the project's protocol, including the issues of informed consent and preservation of privacy and confidentiality. Anonymity was maintained at all times. The subjects were encouraged to ask questions and to address any concerns about the study. Additionally, they had the option to refuse to answer questions that appeared inappropriate to them. Residents with hearing deficits were asked to read the printed material describing the study. The researcher assured the respondents that their responses will not affect their continued care and status at the facility. Questionnaires were designed to maximize confidentiality.

All the eligible residents participated in the project and signed the consent form. Occasionally, the researcher was referred by the residents to family members or significant others to discuss the issue of informed consent. Verbal consent was deemed an acceptable alternative for those residents who were physically unable to provide written permission. In addition, family members were apprised of the goals and content of the project.

Prior to the interview, residents were granted the opportunity to raise questions about the project. The duration of each interview varied between twenty to ninety minutes. Various respondents spoke of their past experiences and substantiated their answers by telling personal stories and exhibiting family pictures. Two residents expressed their wish to terminate the interview and subsequently withdrew their participation from the study.

Following each interview, the researcher retrieved pertinent demographic data from the medical charts along with information about each resident's Activities of Daily Living (ADLs). Upon completion of the data collection, each social worker was asked to assess the adjustment of their clients by responding to an objective scoring questionnaire. Instructions were provided to the workers for this task in order to avoid variations in responses and to increase the reliability of the findings.

RESULTS

Tables 1 and 2 describe the demographic and selected characteristics of the study. The sample was comprised of 77.2 percent female respondents and 22.8 percent male respondents. Religious affiliation among the African American subjects was recorded as 81 percent Protestants/Baptists, 9.5 percent Catholics and 9.5 percent Jehovah's Witnesses. Half of the subjects identified themselves as somewhat religious (50.0 percent). Respondents who rated themselves as very religious comprised 28.3 percent while 21.7 percent possessed a self-perception of not being religious at all. The chi-square test indicated that African-Americans were significantly more religious than their Jewish peers at a $p < .001$ significance level.

Table 2 outlines the mean, standard deviation and t-tests of all religious activities and various sample characteristics by ethnic background. African American residents tended to participate in religious services more frequently than their Jewish peers ($t = 3.03$, $p < .01$). With regard to private displays of religious behavior, the results showed the following:

- Frequency of participation in reading religious material was greater among African American residents ($t = 5.89$, $p < .001$);
- Frequency of private prayer was significantly higher among African American residents ($t = 2.06$, $p < .05$);
- As well as the frequency of watching or listening to a religious program ($t = 2.83$, $p < .01$).

TABLE 1. Comparison of Sample Characteristics by Ethnic Background

Characteristic	Jewish	African American	Total	Chi-square
	(n = 71)	(n = 21)	(N = 92)	
	%	%	%	
Gender				
Male	19.7	33.3	22.8	1.70
Female	80.3	66.7	77.2	
Marital Status				
Widowed	71.8	52.4	67.4	8.28*
Married	8.5	33.3	14.1	
Never married	12.7	9.5	12.0	
Divorced/separated	7.0	4.8	6.5	
Religion				
Jewish	100.0		77.2	92.00***
Catholic		9.5	2.2	
Protestant/Baptist		81.0	18.5	
Jehovah's Witness		9.5	2.2	
Religious Identity				
Very religious	14.1	76.2	28.3	30.94***
Somewhat religious	59.2	19.0	50.0	
Not religious	26.8	4.8	21.7	
Level of Education				
1-6	8.5	19.0	10.9	9.41
7-9	16.9	33.0	20.7	
10-12	47.9	47.6	47.8	
13-16	22.5		17.4	
17+	4.2		3.3	

Note: *p < .05, **p < .01, ***p < .001.

Variations between the groups were also found in the MMSE scores where Jewish residents scored higher than their African American peers ($t = 2.75$, $p < .01$). The extent of dependence on assistance for mobility and other activities of daily living was greater among African Americans than their Jewish peers ($t = 2.62$, $p < .01$). Of the sampled popula-

TABLE 2. Means and T-Tests of Religious Activities and Various Sample Characteristics by Ethnic Background

Characteristic	Jewish		African American		t-value
	M	SD	M	SD	
Frequency of Group Activities					
Attend religious services	3.06	1.57	4.19	1.29	3.03**
Pray in a group	3.04	1.62	3.81	1.47	1.95
Go to church/ synagogue	2.90	1.55	3.62	1.59	1.85
Frequency of Private Activities					
Read the Bible/ religious books	2.35	1.54	4.48	1.08	5.89***
Pray privately	4.06	1.60	4.81	.87	2.06*
Watch/Listen to a religious program	3.08	1.63	4.19	1.36	2.83**
Age (years)	88.14	6.32	81.33	7.77	4.11***
Length of stay (days)	1012.50	1168.40	841.47	614.30	.64
Number of living children	1.25	1.08	1.61	1.69	1.19
Mini-Mental Status Exam	25.24	3.22	23.00	3.48	2.75**
Extent of Dependency on ADLs					
Eating	2.11	.60	2.29	.56	1.18
Mobility	3.01	1.21	3.81	1.25	2.62**
Toileting	2.96	1.18	3.38	1.32	1.41
Transfer	2.63	.72	3.00	.84	1.97

Note: T-test statistics were used. $^*p < .05$, $^{**}p < .01$, $^{***}p < .001$.

tion, Jewish respondents were significantly older than African American respondents (t = 4.11, p < .001). The groups did not vary significantly in their length of stay at the facility, number of living children and level of dependence upon professional staff for eating, toileting and transfer.

Data Reduction

As a preliminary to statistical analysis relating religiosity to adjustment and satisfaction, a data reduction was performed. Many of the variables in Table 2 can be grouped into sets referring to similar characteristics such as ADLs and religiosity. A factor analysis was performed for each set of variables that was considered.

The results showed that the six religious activities in Table 2 and the religious identity value from Table 1 (coded as a three point scale) were all strongly intercorrelated, with a minimum correlation ranging from .337 to .777. The first principal component indicated an eigenvalue of 4.20. It also reflected that the seven items were well summarized by a single factor. The second eigenvalue reached .83, illuminating that it was not the case that the seven items could represent an additional distinction such as group versus private behaviors.

The four ADLs were highly intercorrelated with correlations ranging from .414 to .746. The first principal component had an eigenvalue of 2.70, indicating that the measure of the four ADLs was well summarized by a single factor.

An additional factor analysis was conducted on eight demographic variables including dummy coded variables reflecting marital status. The absolute value of the correlations ranged from .001 to .397. The first principal component had an eigenvalue of 1.84. As these eight variables were not well summarized by factors, they were used separately in the regression analysis.

A factor analysis was performed on eight adjustment items. With four exceptions, the remaining twenty-four correlations ranged from .323 to .776. The first principal component showed an eigenvalue of 4.16; the corresponding correlation with each of the eight items was above .5. Therefore, this principal component was used to summarize the eight adjustment items.

The factor analysis conducted for three social support items delineated social visits, family involvement and telephone conversations with family or significant others. The correlations ranged from .521 to

.630. The first principal component had an eigenvalue of 2.13 and was subsequently used to summarize social support.

The Relationships of Religiosity, Adjustment and Satisfaction

The data reduction yielded a single summary measure of religiosity and a single summary measure of adjustment. These two factors were significantly correlated ($r = .212$, $p = .043$). Religiosity was also significantly correlated with the satisfaction scale–NHRQ ($r = .239$, $p = .022$). Adjustment and satisfaction were also significantly correlated ($r = .257$, $p = .013$).

Stepwise multiple regression analyses were performed to determine whether the relationships of religiosity to adjustment and satisfaction were affected by demographics and other characteristics. The first predictor was ethnic background–Jewish or African American. The second step was eight other demographic variables: gender, age, educational level, living arrangement (private vs. double room), currently married, ever married, number of living children and a self rating of general health. General health was grouped with the demographic variable as it was not associated with any of the other categories. The third step included two measures of functioning–ADL factor and MMSE score. The fourth step included two measures of adjustment to the home, logarithm of the length of stay (transformed to reduce non-normality) and the social support factor.

After all other resident characteristics were examined, the next step involved the religiosity factor. An additional step measured the interaction of religiosity according to ethnic origin. The interaction variable was calculated as the product of the religiosity factor and the ethnic background variable. Inclusion of this interaction in the stepwise analyses after including the ethnic background and the religiosity factor as predictors, tests whether the association of religiosity differs for residents with different ethnic backgrounds.

The results of the stepwise regression analyses predicting the adjustment factor are presented in Table 3. The only step with statistically significant associations is reflected in the demographics. Upon examination of the partial correlations of the demographic predictors of adjustment when controlling for ethnic background, it was revealed that being married was the sole significant value ($r = .278$, $p = .008$). Although the simple correlation of religiosity with adjustment was deemed significant, the partial correlation in controlling for ethnic background, demographics, functioning and social support, was not significant ($r = .172$, $p =$

TABLE 3. Stepwise Multiple Regression Analyses of Selected Independent Variables and Adjustment

Predictors	R^2 change	df1	df2	F	P
Ethnicity	.002	1	90	.165	.686
Demographic	.195	8	82	2.482	.018
Functioning (ADLs and MMSE)	.042	2	80	2.230	.114
Social Support and L.O.S.	.048	2	78	2.639	.078
Religiosity	.021	1	77	2.359	.129
Religiosity × Ethnicity	.000	1	76	.017	.896

Dependent Variable: Resident Adjustment
Note: Demographics = Age, Gender, Married, Ever Married, Living Children, Education, Living Arrangements (single vs. double room) and Good Health.

.13). Additionally, the interaction of ethnic background with religiosity was viewed as insignificant (p = .90).

The results of the stepwise regression analyses predicting the satisfaction of the resident with nursing home living (NHRQ) are presented in Table 4. The sole step of statistical significant association was social support and length of stay. Examination of the partial correlations of controlling for ethnic background, demographics and functioning showed that social support was significant (r = .387, p < .001). Although the simple correlation of religiosity with satisfaction was significant, the partial correlation controlling for ethnic background, demographics, functioning and social support was not significant (r = .146, p = .20). The interaction of ethnic background with religiosity was non-significant (p = .84).

DISCUSSION

The adjustment of a resident to a long-term care facility can be influenced by a myriad of variables. This study examines the association be-

TABLE 4. Stepwise Multiple Regression Analyses of Selected Independent Variables and Satisfaction

Predictors	R^2 change	df1	df2	F	P
Ethnicity	.029	1	90	2.65	.107
Demographic	.092	8	82	1.073	.390
Functioning (ADLs and MMSE)	.026	2	80	1.237	.296
Social Support and L.O.S.	.124	2	78	6.640	.002
Religiosity	.016	1	77	1.674	.200
Religiosity × Ethnicity	.000	1	76	.040	.842

Dependent Variable: Resident Satisfaction (NHRQ)
Note: Demographics = Age, Gender, Married, Ever Married, Living Children, Education, Living Arrangements (single vs. double room) and Good Health.

tween religiosity, adjustment and satisfaction of long term care residents with nursing home living. The findings revealed that the level of religiosity of the individual was significantly associated with resident adjustment and satisfaction. However, after controlling for a variety of other characteristics, these associations were reduced. This conclusion corroborates additional studies that document the connection between level of religiosity and a decrease in depressive symptoms (Musick, Koenig, Hays & Cohen, 1998; Ai, Dunkle, Peterson & Bolling, 1998), as well as an increase in morale, sense of usefulness and quality of life (Ellison & Gay, 1990; Koenig, Kvale & Ferrel, 1988).

The study illustrates the importance of controlling for select characteristics. The simple examination of the results shows that religiosity is significantly associated with the adjustment and satisfaction of the resident, yet, after controlling for other variables, the association was reduced. While other studies document the predictive power of demographic variables with nursing home resident adjustment and satisfaction, this study did not reach a similar conclusion. It is possible that differences between the sample populations in other studies such as a younger mean age, a higher level of functioning of the subjects and/or a shorter length of stay at the facility contribute to the predictive power of these variables. Other independent variables targeted as strongly correlated with resident satisfaction include the extent of family involvement, desire to relocate to the nursing home and being married.

Several theories are offered to support the positive association between level of religiosity and resident satisfaction. Residents who exhibit a high level of religiosity may sense that their quality of life will improve at the nursing home through a continued involvement in religious activities, thus, generating greater peer interaction and mutual support. Additionally as suggested by Ellison (1994), involvement in religious activities may reduce the rate and risk of exposure to certain stressors that are generally associated with nursing home living. Hence, future research endeavors may inspect the link between religious factors, and their effect on social stressors, and the well-being of nursing home residents.

Engagement in private religious activities can create an opportunity to ventilate concerns, feelings and hopes for the future. The distinction of private prayer as the most prevalent religious activity may stem from the elder's ability to find comfort through a personal connection with God. Moreover, the act of prayer can be practiced at all times and does not require any prior preparation, knowledge or special abilities in order to be effective. It is therefore likely that an increased sense of inner tranquility will affect the individual's ability to cope positively in the new environment. The findings did not corroborate a link between ethnic affiliation and level of satisfaction. Therefore, Jewish residents were not found to be significantly more or less satisfied with nursing home living than their African American counterparts. However, African American residents perceived themselves as significantly more religious than their Jewish peers. Therefore, the interdisciplinary team's challenge is to develop a spiritual atmosphere that is sensitive to their diverse needs and religious practices.

The main limitation of the study involves the selection of the sample. The convenience sample was chosen with several predetermined criteria due to the availability of the subjects and their capacity to respond to the questions. Additionally, the proportion of African American residents was smaller than their Jewish peers. The home consists of primarily Jewish and secondarily, African American residents. Thus, it did not include other religious groups. This impacts upon the generalization of the findings to the entire nursing home population. Hence, future research should examine these questions among other ethnic and religious groups. This study can serve as a springboard for other studies of this population.

Additionally, the resident population diagnosed with a level of moderate to severe dementia (scored below 20 on MMSE) was excluded from participating in the study due to their cognitive limitations. New methods of inquiry and assessment can be developed to evaluate the level of religiosity and subsequent adjustment process of these residents as well. Further exploration of this special group is primary to all studies on aging as involvement in spiritual and religious activities can be meaningful, stimulating and non-threatening to cognitively impaired residents as well.

Despite the limitations, the findings of the study may be useful for social work clinicians in many heterogeneous and culturally diverse nursing homes. The preservation of a religious identity within the institutional environment appears to maintain the well-being of older adults. This can be accomplished by creating mechanisms through which residents can maintain their cultural roles and religious practices. Clinicians can utilize their knowledge, skills and expertise to assess the multiple facets comprising a resident's level of religiosity. Key factors to be considered include the adult's support system, values, norms, patterns of interdependency, previous roles, spiritual and cultural practices (formal and informal).

Moreover, the function of religious role in the long term care environment can be a powerful healing device to shield the anguish of illness, loss and multiple changes incurred by this major life transition. A detailed plan of care for each resident should encompass a comprehensive assessment of religious needs, level of celebration of religious holidays and ritual, role of prayer in the individual's life, the extent of involvement in church or synagogue and ethnic and cultural preferences. Finally, enabling the continuation of previous religious roles, activities and behavior and attempting to fulfill the spiritual needs of nursing home residents would likely prompt increased satisfaction and a more successful adjustment to the long-term care setting.

REFERENCES

Abramowitz, L. (1993). Prayer as therapy among the frail Jewish elderly. *Journal of Gerontological Social Work, 19,* (3/4), 69-75.

Ai, A.M., Dunkle, R.E., Peterson, C. & Bolling, S.F. (1998). The role of private prayer in psychological recovery among midlife and aged patients following cardiac surgery. *The Gerontologist, 38*(5), 591-601.

Amen, A.M. (1959). Informal groups and institutional adjustment in a Catholic home for the aging. *Journal of Gerontology, 14*, 338-343.

Ames, D. (1991). Epidemiological studies of depression among the elderly in residential and nursing homes. *International Journal of Geriatric Psychiatry, 6*, 347-354.

Blazer, D. & Palmore, E. (1976). Religion and aging in a longitudinal panel. *The Gerontologist, 16*(1), 82-85.

Butler, R.N. (1985). *Why survive? Being old in America.* New York: Harper & Row.

Chatters, L.M. & Taylor, R.J. (1989). Age differences in religious participation among Black adults. *Journal of Gerontology: Social Sciences, 44*(5), 183-189.

Cohen, C.I., Hyland, K. & Magai, C. (1998). Interracial and intraracial differences in neuropsychiatric symptoms, sociodemography and treatment among nursing home patients with dementia. *The Gerontologist, 38*(3), 353-361.

Dick, H.R. & Friedsam, H.J. (1963). Adjustment of residents of two homes for the aged. *Social Problems, 11*, 282-290.

Ellison, C.G. (1994). Religion, the life stress paradigm and the study of depression. In J.S. Levin (Ed.), *Religion in aging and health.* Thousand Oaks, CA: Sage Publications.

Ellison, C.G. & Gay, D.A. (1990). Religion, religious commitment and life satisfaction among black Americans. *The Sociological Quarterly, 31*(1), 123-147.

Folstein, M. F., Folstein, S. & McHugh, P.R. (1975). "Mini-Mental State": A practical method for grading the cognitive state of patients for the clinician. *Journal of Psychiatric Research, 12*, 189-198.

Husaini, B.A., Blasi, A.J. & Miller, O. (1999). Does public and private religiosity have a moderating effect on depression? A bi-racial study of elders in the American south. *International Journal of Aging and Human Development, 48*(1), 63-72.

Jacobson, C.K., Heaton, T.B. & Dennis, R.M. (1990). Black-White differences in religiosity: Item analyses and a formal structural test. *Sociological Analysis, 51*(3), 257-270.

Johnson, B.D., Stone, G.L., Altmaier, E.M. & Berdahl, L.D. (1998). The relationship of demographic factors, locus of control and self-efficacy to successful nursing home adjustment. *The Gerontologist, 38*(2), 209-216.

Joiner, C.M. (1989). *Factors in nursing home adjustment and satisfaction.* Unpublished doctoral dissertation. Washington, DC: Washington University.

Joiner, C.M. & Freudiger, P.T. (1993). Male and female differences in nursing home adjustment and satisfaction. *Journal of Gerontological Social Work, 20*(3/4), 71-85.

Kane, R., Riegler, S., Bell, R., Potter, R. & Koshland, G. (1982). *Predicting the course of nursing home patients: A progress report.* CA: The Rand Corporation.

Koenig, H.G., Kvale, J. N. & Ferrel, C. (1988). Religion and well-being in later life. *The Gerontologist, 28*(1), 18-27.

Koenig, H.G., Smiley, M. & Gonzales, J.A. (1988). *Religion, health and aging.* New York: Greenwood Press.

Koenig, H.G., Cohen, H.J., Blazer, D.G., Pieper, C., Meador, K.G., Shelp, F., Goli, V. & DiPasquale, B. (1992). Religious coping and depression among elderly, hospitalized medically ill men. *The American Journal of Psychiatry, 149*(12), 1693-1700.

Koenig, H.G., George, L.K. & Peterson, B.L. (1998). Religiosity and remission of depression in medically ill older patients. *The American Journal of Psychiatry*, *155*(4), 536-542.

Larson, D.B., Donahue, M.J., Lyons, J.S., Benson, P.L., Pattison, M., Worthington, E.L. & Blazer, D.G. (1989). Religious affiliations in mental health research samples as compared with national samples. *Journal of Nervous and Mental Disease*, *177*(2), 109-111.

Levin, J.S. & Taylor, R.J. (1997). Age differences in patterns and correlates of the frequency of prayer. *The Gerontologist*, *37*(1), 75-88.

Levin, J.S., Chatters, L.M. & Taylor, R.J. (1995). Religious effects on health status and life satisfaction among Black Americans. *Journal of Gerontology: Social Sciences*, *50B*(3), S154-S163.

Markides, K.S., Levin, J.S. & Ray, L. (1987). Religion, aging, and life satisfaction: An eight-year, three-wave longitudinal study. *The Gerontologist*, *27*(5), 660-665.

Moberg, D.O. (1970). Religion in the later years. In A. M. Hoffman (Ed.). *The daily needs and interests of older persons*. Illinois: Charles C. Thomas.

Mui, C.A. & Burnette, D. (1994). Long-term care service use by frail elders: Is ethnicity a factor? *The Gerontologist*, *34*(2), 190-198.

Mull, C.S., Cox, C. L. & Sullivan, J.A. (1987). Religion's role in the health and well-being of well elders. *Public Health Nursing*, *4*(3), 151-159.

Musick, M.A., Koenig, H.G., Hays, J.C. & Cohen, H.J. (1998). Religious activity and depression among community-dwelling elderly persons with cancer: The moderating effect of race. *Journal of Gerontology: Social Sciences*, *53B*(4), S218-S227.

Redfoot, D.L. (1987). On the separtin' place: Social class and relocation among older women. *Social Forces*, *66*(2), 486-500.

Rodstein, M., Savitsky, E. & Starkman, R. (1976). Initial adjustment to a long-term care institution: Medical and behavioral aspects. *Journal of the American Geriatric Society*, *24*(2), 65-71.

Schiller, P.L. & Levin, J.S. (1988). Is there a religious factor in health care utilization? A review. *Social Science and Medicine*, *27*(12), 1369-79.

Shanas, E. (1979). The family as a social support system in old age. *The Gerontologist*, *19*(2), 169-174.

Sigman, S.J. (1986). Adjustment to the nursing home as a social interactional accomplishment. *Journal of Applied Communication Research*, *14*(1), 37-58.

Stolley, J.M. & Koenig, H. (1997). Religion/Spirituality and health among elderly African Americans and Hispanics. *Journal of Psychosocial Nursing*, *35*(11), 32-38.

Tobin, S.S. (1995). Fostering family involvement in institutional care. In G.C. Smith, S. S. Tobin, E.A., Robertson-Tchabo & P. W. Power (Eds.). *Strengthening aging families: Diversity in practice and policy*. CA: Sage Publications, Inc.

Physical Dysfunction and Social Participation Among Racial/Ethnic Groups of Older Americans: Implications for Social Work

Elizabeth M. Bertera
Barbara Bailey-Etta

SUMMARY. This paper reports the findings of a study that was undertaken to (1) identify differences in social participation patterns among racial/ethnic and gender groups, (2) examine the association between physical dysfunction and church and club attendance, and (3) explore opportunities for social work interventions that improve the quality of life of older Americans. The study was based on a national sample representative of the 39 million Americans age 60 and over.

The data indicate that those who attended both church and club meetings had the lowest levels of physical dysfunction; those who attended one but not the other had intermediate levels of dysfunction, and those who did not attend church and also did not attend club meetings had the highest dysfunction levels. These findings suggest that physical limita-

---

Elizabeth M. Bertera is affiliated with the Catholic University of America, Shahan Hall, Washington, DC 20064.

Barbara Bailey-Etta is affiliated with the Catholic University of America, Shahan Hall, Washington, DC 20064.

This study was supported in part by a grant-in-aid from the Catholic University of America in Washington, DC.

[Haworth co-indexing entry note]: "Physical Dysfunction and Social Participation Among Racial/Ethnic Groups of Older Americans: Implications for Social Work." Bertera, Elizabeth M., and Barbara Bailey-Etta. Co-published simultaneously in *Social Thought* (The Haworth Press, Inc.) Vol. 20, No. 3/4, 2001, pp. 97-115; and: *Issues in Global Aging* (ed: Frederick L. Ahearn, Jr.) The Haworth Press, Inc., 2001, pp. 97-115. Single or multiple copies of this article are available for a fee from The Haworth Document Delivery Service [1-800-HAWORTH, 9:00 a.m. - 5:00 p.m. (EST). E-mail address: getinfo@haworthpressinc.com].

tions reduce participation in social activities at church and in clubs, which may limit access to social support for older persons that could benefit the most from it. Social workers should seek ways of identifying natural support systems when working with older adults to help provide social participation opportunities for older persons, especially those that may have access and mobility problems due to physical limitations. *[Article copies available for a fee from The Haworth Document Delivery Service: 1-800-HAWORTH. E-mail address: <getinfo@haworthpressinc.com> Website: <http://www.HaworthPress.com>* © *2001 by The Haworth Press, Inc. All rights reserved.]*

KEYWORDS. Older adults, social support, participation, physical dysfunction, church attendance, club affiliation

INTRODUCTION

Despite the lack of consensus in defining, operationalizing, and measuring social support as a positive force in the lives of the elderly, a number of consistent findings emerge. Social support can be given and received (Bertera, 1997) and it is important to health and well-being, particularly for aging adults (Antonucci, Ajrouch, & Janevic, 1999; Forster & Stoller, 1992). Older adults with few social ties have increased risk of dying earlier, whereas those with social support have a survival advantage. Older adults who see themselves as socially engaged and supported are in better mental and physical health than those socially isolated (Siebert, Mutran, & Reitzes, 1999). Gerontological researchers are interested in social support mechanisms because of their potential usefulness in the care, health maintenance, and sustained independence of older adults. Social support can be formal or informal. For the purposes of this study, social support is defined as an informal, social participation that occurs as part of natural support, which includes a network of individuals represented by attendance at church and membership in social club groups in the community. The nature and the sources of social support have undergone considerable change in recent years. The greater separation of adult children from their older parents, full employment and the austerity in government funding of social service programs have forced many older adults to turn to the church and clubs for social affiliation and support.

Social support as measured by church attendance has been positively associated with health status and life satisfaction among older adults (Auslander, 1988; Barusch, 1999; Berg, Fonss, Reed, & VandeCreek, 1995; Darrow, Russell, Cooper, Mudar, & Frone, 1992; Fox, Pitkin, Paul, Carson, & Duan, 1998; Guy, 1982; Heisel & Faulkner, 1982; Markides, 1983; Suarez, Lloyd, Weiss, Rainbolt, & Pulley, 1994; Young & Dowling, 1987). Among the various methods of measuring a person's religiosity, perhaps one of the most often used is church attendance. Church attendance by different religious groups was found to be 66% for Catholics, 46% for Protestants and 25% for Jews (Cox, 1993). A number of scientists have observed the potentially positive value that religious faith and activities can have on the lives of older Americans. The psychological supports that religion provides older persons help them to: (1) find and maintain a sense of meaningfulness and significance in life; (2) accept the inevitable losses of old age; and (3) discover and utilize the compensatory values that are potential in old age; and (4) face impending death (Cox, 1993). Religious institutions often provide a number of social functions that can be particularly useful for older Americans. For example, they provide a variety of social activities that bring people of all ages and backgrounds together. The social affiliation that ensues tends to increase interaction and reduce the individual's social isolation. The interest shown for older adults by other individuals in church or clubs becomes a source of social support that may lead to changes in social interactions, awareness of services, health behaviors and even health status.

The link between physical dysfunction and social participation as measured by church and club attendance has also generated research. A decline in functional status has been associated with reduction in frequency of church attendance but not with any change in rates of religious media use (TV/radio) (Guy, 1982; Idler & Kasl, 1997). Research on disabilities and participation suggest an association between activity limitations and social participation among not only older adults but also younger populations (Campbell, Crews, Moriarty, Zack, & Blackman, 1999; Daly & Berman, 1993; Dijkers, 1999; Fried, Bandeen-Roche, Kasper, & Guralnik, 1999; Whitehouse, Shope, Sullivan, & Kulik, 1989). However, research on the interactions of race/ethnicity, gender, physical dysfunction and social participation are limited.

This paper will examine social participation as measured by church and club attendance among older Americans. The purpose is to (1) identify differences in social participation patterns among racial/ethnic and gender groups, (2) examine the association between physical dysfunction and church and club attendance, and (3) explore opportunities for social work interventions that improve the quality of life of older Americans.

RELEVANCE

There have been relatively few studies on social participation as measured by church and club attendance in large population samples. Older adults often turn to religious organizations, rely on religious beliefs and social supports to help them in coping with routine challenges of daily life and hardships resulting from severe adversity (Barusch, 1999). Moreover, previous research has pointed out that religion plays an important role in life satisfaction of older Americans. However, there has been limited research conducted on examining the association between church attendance, club attendance and physical dysfunction among older Americans.

A number of authors have posited that church attendance and social clubs are measures of life satisfaction for older Americans (Allen-Meares, 1995; Barusch, 1999; Carter, 2000; Daley, 1995; Delgado, 1996; Guy, 1982; Heisel & Faulkner, 1982; Koenig, Bearon, Hover, & Travis, 1991; Ortega, 1983). Guy (1982) conducted a study on the role of older age cohorts with emphasis on life satisfaction relative to age, physical disabilities, and church attendance. A significant finding was that there is strong relationship between church attendance and life satisfaction. Further, while church attendance may decrease with age as physical activity limitations increase, the elderly will have more life satisfaction if they maintain social contact at church and clubs (Guy, 1982).

The church has historically played a unique role in the African American and Latino communities (Heisel & Faulkner, 1982). Markides (1983), Boyd-Franklin (1989), and Holmes and Holmes (1995) state that African Americans and Latinos throughout history have regarded the church as a haven and the only institution that belonged exclusively to their community (Holmes & Holmes, 1995). However, the role of the church in the lives of these groups has yielded limited empirical research. For example, Heisel and Faulkner (1982) interviewed 122 urban African Americans between the ages of 51-90. Using Glock's conceptual framework, they found that religiosity remained stable over the later years. However, it appeared to become more significant in the life of an older person when other activities and involvement lessened, e.g., retirement, widowhood and reduction of parental responsibilities. It was found that church membership did vary with age, women had higher scores than men and that "religiosity was positively related to life satisfaction and to frequency of church attendance regardless of age and sex" (Heisel & Faulkner, 1982).

Billingsley (1992) reflects that approximately 70% of African Americans attend church and when they are no longer able to attend, they still consider themselves parishioners. Church plays a central role in African-American families and in the community. In a later article, Carter (2000) stated that it is through the African American Church that relationship is kindled, political advocacy is extolled, isolation is decreased and positive interaction occurs.

Markides, in a longitudinal analysis of aging, religiosity and adjustment among Mexican-Americans and Anglos, used three indicators of religiosity: church attendance, self-rated religiosity, and practice of private prayer. He sought to examine: (1) whether there was any evidence of increase or decline with aging in church attendance, self-rated religiosity, and practice of private prayer; (2) whether the religious variables are related positively to life satisfaction (net of other important predictors of adjustment); and (3) whether these relationships increase with time (Markides, 1983). Probability, random sampling was used and 510 adults were interviewed. The mean age was 69.8 with 70% Mexican-Americans and 30% Anglos. Women comprised 60% of the group. Findings disclosed women to be more religious than men; more Mexican-Americans were Catholic, partial support for the hypothesis relating religiosity with aging over time. Significant was the finding that church attendance was the only religious variable positively related to life satisfaction (Markides, 1983).

Delgado (1996), in his article on religion as a caregiving system, noted that there is a scarcity of articles examining the role of religion in the lives of Puerto Rican elders in the United States. He related that the Hartford study remains one of the few published research efforts in this area and the findings were as follows:

> (1) Faith is viewed as a critical element in an elder's life; (2) Puerto Rican elders were not attending church as often compared with previous years (8 percent); (3) Females consider themselves more religious than males; (4) One percent consider themselves very religious compared to 23 percent for males. Religion as a support system increases its significance for Puerto Rican elders who have left Puerto Rico and settled in the United States, finding

themselves increasingly more isolated from family and community. (Delgado, 1996)

In summary, these studies show a positive correlation between religion and life satisfaction, attitudes, values and beliefs that help older persons evaluate and understand the world around them (Markides, 1983; Ortega et al., 1983; Billingsley, 1992; Cox, 1993; Carter, 2000). Moreover, attendance at church helps older persons affiliate with religious activities and obtain social support (Barusch, 1999; Billingsley, 1992; Carter, 2000; Cox, 1993). Studies have also shown that when older adults are no longer able to attend church, they still consider themselves members and in some instances continue to receive social support (Billingsley, 1992).

METHODOLOGY

The data for this study were obtained from an existing database collected in the National Health and Nutrition Examination Survey (NHANES III) 1988 through 1994 (U.S. Dept. Health and Human Services, July 1997). The NHANES III was a national representative cross-sectional survey with an in-person interview, medical examination and lab tests of non-institutionalized persons in the United States aged 17 and older. The general structure of the NHANES III sample design was similar to that of previous NHANES: Complex, multi-stage, and stratified, clustered samples of civilian non-institutionalized populations were used. After NHANES recommended weights were applied, the study sample of 6529 was weighted to represent a population estimate of 39 million persons age 60 and over.

Social participation was measured by church attendance and club affiliation. Church attendance was measured by the specific question: How often do you attend church or religious services? Church attendance was operationalized by dichotomizing the responses as follows: attended church one or more times in the past year versus did not attend in past year. Club membership was measured by the question: How often do you attend meetings of the clubs or organizations you belong to? Dichotomizing the responses as follows operationalized club membership: attended one or more club meetings in the last year versus did not attend any meetings.

Physical dysfunction was measured by responses to 17 items that may cause limitations due to health or physical problems: walking a quarter mile, walking up 10 steps, stooping/kneeling, lifting 10 pounds, doing household chores, preparing meals, walking from room to room, standing up in an armless chair, getting out of bed, eating/cutting food, dressing, personal care, handling routines, using a device to get around, using special utensils, using aids to get dressed. All items had response choices/scores as follows: No Difficulty (0), Some Difficulty (1), Much Difficulty (2), Unable to Do (3). Physical dysfunction index scores ranged from 0, indicating no physical disability to 39, indicating a high degree of difficulty with daily activities. Index development for the physical dysfunction items yielded a Cronbach Alpha of .88. This indicates an acceptable level of internal consistency among the 17 items in the Index.

Bivariate analyses were conducted to describe the sociodemographic characteristics of the sample and to examine relationships among the variables. Associations among categorical variables were tested for statistical significance using chi-square. The complex relationships among the independent and dependent variables were investigated by regression techniques. Using a MANOVA approach, regression was used to test hypotheses in which physical functioning was the dependent variable, church and club attendance were independent variables, and racial/ethnic group and gender were factor variables used to separate the study population into subgroups for more detailed analysis.

FINDINGS

The study population consisted of persons 60 years of age and older. They were predominantly white (86 percent), African American (8.5 percent), Other Hispanics (3 percent) and Mexican-Americans (2.3 percent) as shown in Table 1. A somewhat higher proportion of the population was female (57.4 percent) compared with male. Within racial-ethnic groups the highest percent female was in the Other Hispanic group. The majority of the study population was in the 60 to 74 age group, with the Mexican-American and Other Hispanic groups showing the youngest age structure. The vast majority of the sample consisted of married individuals with the spouse or partner living in the home. This was highest among the Mexican-American and white respondents with about 60 percent each and lowest among Other Hispanics and African Americans. In addition, marital status among African American respondents indicated the highest percent of widows (see Table 1).

ISSUES IN GLOBAL AGING

TABLE 1. Socio-Demographic Characteristics by Racial/Ethnic Group

Characteristic	White	African American	Mexican- American	Other Hispanic	Totals	X^2 (df, p value)
Weighted Number Totals	33,831,267	3,343,773	914,703	1,198,945	39,288,688	
Percent Totals	86.1	8.5	2.3	3.1	100.0	
Male	43.0	40.3	45.2	35.6	42.6	**36762** (3, < .001)
Female	57.0	59.7	54.8	64.4	57.4	
Age 60 - 74	69.9	73.2	82.3	81.3	70.8	**145524** (3, < .001)
75 or more	30.1	26.8	17.7	18.7	29.2	
Married/Living as married	63.0	43.0	64.7	52.7	61.1	
Widowed	26.6	39.3	22.9	22.2	27.3	
Divorced	5.8	8.5	5.6	14.7	6.3	**123527** (12, < .001)
Separated	.6	4.9	3.0	4.7	1.2	
Never married	4.0	4.3	3.8	5.7	4.1	
8 years or less	20.4	44.6	71.5	46.1	24.4	
9 - 11 years	17.0	20.3	11.1	5.1	16.8	**268139** (9, < .001)
High school	32.2	21.1	10.8	30.4	30.7	
College or more	30.4	14.0	6.6	18.4	28.1	
$10,000 or less	14.5	36.1	27.9	21.6	16.9	
$11,000-$19,000	26.6	26.0	31.4	24.3	26.6	**123143** (9, < .001)
$20,000-$39,000	29.1	17.2	19.0	29.6	27.8	
$40,000 or more	29.8	20.7	21.7	24.5	28.7	

Note: All characteristics are reported as column percents.

The educational attainment of the sample differed widely, with more than three-quarters of the Mexican-American respondents reporting less than a high school education, compared with about two-thirds of African Americans and only one-third of whites. Family income also varied with approximately 43 percent of all respondents indicating family income of less than $20,000 per year. Nearly two-thirds of African Americans reported incomes less than $20,000 per year, followed by Mexican-Americans, Other Hispanics and whites (see Table 1).

Social Participation

Church participation, defined as attending church at least once during the past year, was higher for females compared with males for all racial/ethnic groups except Other Hispanics (see Table 2). Among males, church attendance was highest among Other Hispanics, followed by African Americans, Mexican-Americans and whites, in that order. Among females, the highest rate of church attendance was found among African Americans, followed by Mexican-Americans, whites and Other Hispanics.

Another measure of social participation was attendance at club meetings at least once each year (see Table 2, lower half). Compared with church attendance, club attendance did not vary as much between male and female respondents. However, club attendance was slightly higher for females compared to males for African American and Other Hispanic respondents. The reverse was observed among white and Mexican-American respondents where males were slightly more likely to

TABLE 2. Church Attendance and Club Membership by Racial/Ethnic Group

Affiliation	White	African American	Mexican-American	Other Hispanic	Total	X^2 (df, p value)
Church attendance						
Male**						
Yes	57.6%	67.8%	67.7%	81.2%	59.3	**154819**
No	42.4%	32.2%	32.3%	18.8%	40.7	(3, < .001)
Total	100.0%	100.0%	100.0%	100.0%	100.0%	
Female**						**231050**
Yes	69.7%	84.9%	80.7%	67.4%	71.2	(3, < .001)
No	30.3%	15.1%	19.3%	32.6%	28.8	
Total	100.0%	100.0%	100.0%	100.0%	100.0%	
Club membership						
Male**						
Yes	48.8%	28.9%	14.7%	19.1%	45.6	
No	51.2%	71.1%	85.3%	80.9%	54.4	**490141**
Total	100.0%	100.0%	100.0%	100.0%	100.0%	(3, < .001)
Female**						
Yes	45.3%	32.2%	11.5%	23.8%	42.6	
No	54.7%	67.8%	88.5%	76.2%	57.4	**454453**
Total	100.0%	100.0%	100.0%	100.0%	100.0%	(3, < .001)

attend clubs compared with females. For both male and female respondents, whites were by far the most likely to attend clubs, followed by African Americans, Other Hispanics and Mexican-Americans (see Table 2).

The overall pattern of social participation found in the bivariate analysis is complex. For both Hispanic males and African American males, there is a strong tendency to report church attendance more than club attendance; however, for white males, church attendance and club membership are more closely matched. For Mexican-American females and African American females, there is a pronounced tendency to report more church attendance than club attendance, while for Other Hispanic females and white females, the same tendency is observed but with not as strong a commitment to church attendance over club membership (see Table 2).

Physical Dysfunction and Social Participation

The adjusted mean physical dysfunction scores and R square results from the regression analysis are shown in Table 3 for main effects and for two-, three- and four-way interactions. Higher dysfunction scores indicate more self-reported limitations in physical activity for the 17 items in the survey. As indicated by the main effects portion of the analysis, greater physical dysfunction was associated with Mexican-American and African American racial/ethnic group, female gender, not attending church and not attending clubs.

As shown in Table 3, the mean dysfunction score was higher for females, regardless of racial/ethnic group and was highest for Mexican-American females, followed by african american females. those reporting no church attendance or no club attendance had mean dysfunction scores higher than those who did attend, regardless of racial/ethnic group. Similarly, those reporting no club attendance or no church attendance had mean dysfunction scores higher than those who did attend, regardless of gender. The three-way interactions, show in the lower half of Table 3, indicate that males who attended church had the lowest dysfunction scores while females who did not attend had the highest physical dysfunction scores. This relationship was consistent within each racial/ethnic group, although within each participation category minority group respondents and females generally had higher mean dysfunction scores compared to whites or males, respectively. The same findings were seen for club attendance, with the exception of Mexican-American females, where those attending club meetings had slightly

TABLE 3. Main Effects and Interaction Effects of Race, Gender, Church Attendance and Club Meeting Attendance by Physical Dysfunction Level

		Estimated Means	R Square
Main Effects			
White		2.9	
African American		3.9	
Mexican-American		4.1	.007
Other Hispanics		2.3	
Male		2.2	
Female		4.3	.020
Attended Church		2.6	
Did Not Attend		3.9	.012
Attended Club Meetings		2.3	
Did Not Attend		4.3	.014
Two-Way Interactions			
White	Male	2.0	
	Female	3.8	
African American	Male	3.3	
	Female	4.5	
Mexican-American	Male	2.3	
	Female	5.9	.015
Other Hispanics	Male	1.5	
	Female	3.1	
White	Attended Church	2.3	
	Did Not Attend	3.5	
African American	Attended Church	3.4	
	Did Not Attend	4.4	
Mexican-American	Attended Church	3.0	
	Did Not Attend	5.2	.012
Other Hispanics	Attended Church	1.8	
	Did Not Attend	2.7	
White	Attended Clubs	2.4	
	Did Not Attend	3.3	
African American	Attended Clubs	1.7	
	Did Not Attend	6.0	
Mexican-American	Attended Clubs	4.6	.013
	Did Not Attend	3.5	
Other Hispanics	Attended Clubs	0.5	
	Did Not Attend	4.1	
Male	Attended Church	1.9	
	Did Not Attend	2.5	
Female	Attended Church	3.3	.000
	Did Not Attend	5.3	
Male	Attended Clubs	1.6	
	Did Not Attend	2.9	
Female	Attended Clubs	3.0	.004
	Did Not Attend	5.6	

TABLE 3 (continued)

		Three-Way Interactions	Estimated Means	R Square
White	Male	Attended Church	1.6	
		Did Not Attend	2.3	
	Female	Attended Church	2.9	
		Did Not Attend	4.6	
African American	Male	Attended Church	2.4	
		Did Not Attend	4.1	
	Female	Attended Church	4.3	
		Did Not Attend	4.7	
Mexican-American	Male	Attended Church	2.5	.003
		Did Not Attend	2.0	
	Female	Attended Church	3.5	
		Did Not Attend	8.3	
Other Hispanics	Male	Attended Church	1.2	
		Did Not Attend	1.7	
	Female	Attended Church	2.5	
		Did Not Attend	3.8	
White	Male	Attended Club Mtg	1.6	
		Did Not Attend	2.3	
	Female	Attended Club Mtg	3.2	
		Did Not Attend	4.3	
African American	Male	Attended Club Mtg	1.9	
		Did Not Attend	4.6	
	Female	Attended Club Mtg	1.5	
		Did Not Attend	7.5	
Mexican-American	Male	Attended Club Mtg	2.7	.000
		Did Not Attend	1.9	
	Female	Attended Club Mtg	6.6	
		Did Not Attend	5.1	
Other Hispanics	Male	Attended Club Mtg	0.0	
		Did Not Attend	2.9	
	Female	Attended Club Mtg	0.9	
		Did Not Attend	5.3	

		Four-Way Interactions		Estimated Means	R Square
		CHURCH	CLUB MEETINGS		
White	Male	Attended	Attended	1.7	
			Did Not Attend	1.6	
		Did Not Attend	Attended	1.6	
			Did Not Attend	3.0	
	Female	Attended	Attended	2.6	
			Did Not Attend	3.3	
		Did Not Attend	Attended	3.8	
			Did Not Attend	5.3	
African American	Male	Attended	Attended	1.9	
			Did Not Attend	2.9	
		Did Not Attend	Attended	1.9	
			Did Not Attend	6.2	
	Female	Attended	Attended	2.9	
			Did Not Attend	5.7	
		Did Not Attend	Attended	0.0	
			Did Not Attend	9.3	

		Four-Way Interactions		Estimated Means	R Square
		CHURCH	CLUB MEETINGS		
Mexican American	Male	Attended	Attended	3.4	.001
			Did Not Attend	1.7	
		Did Not Attend	Attended	2.0	
			Did Not Atend	2.1	
	Female	Attended	Attended	3.1	
			Did Not Attend	3.9	
		Did Not Attend	Attended	10.0	
			Did Not Attend	6.5	
Other Hispanics	Male	Attended	Attended	0.0	
			Did Not Attend	2.4	
		Did Not Attend	Attended	0.0	
			Did Not Attend	3.4	
	Female	Attended	Attended	0.9	
			Did Not Attend	4.0	
		Did Not Attend	Attended	1.0	
			Did Not Attend	6.6	
Grand Mean				3.3	.065

higher dysfunction scores than those who did not attend (6.6 vs. 5.1). These findings suggest that social participation is highest among respondents who had the least amount of physical dysfunction.

The four-way interactions reflect the relationships among racial/ethnic, gender and social participation variables combined as shown at the bottom of Table 3. Those who attended both church and club meetings had the lowest physical dysfunction and those who attended neither church nor club meetings had the highest physical dysfunction. The only exception to this pattern was Mexican-American males, where the mean physical dysfunction score was somewhat higher for those who attended both compared to those who attended neither (3.4 vs. 2.1). The greatest predictor of physical dysfunction was gender, followed by club and church participation, as shown in the R Square column of Table 3. Overall, the study findings indicate that social participation in activities that may be an important source of social support, such as church attendance and club meetings, is limited by physical dysfunction in this sample of older adults.

IMPLICATIONS FOR SOCIAL WORK

This study identified complex patterns of church and club attendance that varied by racial/ethnic group, gender and degree of physical dysfunction. The interaction of the variables supports previous research on the association between participation and disability. In addition, longitudinal research (Idler, 1997) suggests that attendance at church services is a strong predictor of better functioning, even when intermediate changes in functioning are included and that health practices, social ties, and indicators of well-being reduce but do not eliminate these effects. Social participation through activities such as church and club attendance is important for elders because it provides an important source of social support. If social participation declines over time due to the decrease in physical dysfunction, those elders who could benefit the most may be cut off from important sources of social support, which in themselves may contribute to physical and mental health and quality of life. It is essential to seek ways of reducing the effects of physical dysfunction in this population in order to maintain elders access to social support. One important goal for an aging society is to minimize the impact of chronic disease and impairment on the health status of older adults, maintain their ability to live independently, and improve their quality of life. Life satisfaction and quality of life have been linked with physical dysfunction and social participation (Dagnam & Ruddick, 1998; Dijkers, 1999; Gottlieb, 1985; Heath & Fentem, 1997). One limitation of this study is the cross-sectional nature of the data collection. Further research is warranted to examine how quality of life is affected by physical dysfunction and by social participation. This research should use prospective techniques that enable researchers to explore relationships among these variables that may change during the aging process.

Current and future employment of social workers includes a host of settings that serve older populations. Social workers need to find policy and program mechanisms that will enable elders to maintain social participation over time. These policy and program interventions may be directed both at the sources of dysfunction as well as the access that elders have to social participation at church and clubs. There are a variety of policies and programs that could improve health and mobility for elders who are beginning to experience physical dysfunction. These include access to appropriately designed housing, transportation and building access. Other issues could include creative ways of reducing the need for physical mobility such as church services outside of churches, club meetings closer to home, and new social participation opportunities in local neighborhoods specifically designed to address the needs of vulnerable seniors who could benefit the most from undiminished social support. The integration of spirituality and religion in social work practice is consistent with the profession's historical view of the nature of the person holistically and in tune with the bio-psycho-social-spiritual perspective (Joseph, 1988). Retrenchment in social service programs and budget cuts will necessitate turning to other sources to aid in the maintenance and independence of older adults. These factors, coupled with the growth of the elderly population, should prompt social workers to seek out networks of skilled helpers. These helpers could include the church, pastoral counseling and social clubs. Moreover, since the church is considered a "natural support system" that has a great influence on elderly persons' help-seeking behaviors, the church can be involved in assisting with organizing networks and programs to assist the elderly. Church and club attendance could be considered an adjunct to social work interventions with this population. It must be noted that key values in social work require that such programs maintain respect for the uniqueness of the individual elderly person, recognize his/her underlying personality structure, history of life experience, current resources, support networks and religious orientation.

The results of this analysis suggest a strong consistent association between social participation as measured by church attendance and club attendance and in the self-reported level of physical dysfunction experienced by persons age 60 and above. The relationship observed was statistically significant, additive and graduated as indicated in Table 3. However, the cross-sectional nature of the data makes it impossible to establish causality among the variables of interest. Further research is needed in studies that track the same variables in a representative sample over time.

Based on our findings, we propose that the church and clubs be used in a more creative and integrated way in the provision of services to the elderly at both the micro and macro levels. The inclusion of social network intervention training in social welfare could better equip social workers working with the elderly. Seven types of network interventions could be used when working with the elderly according to Froland et al. (1981): Clinical Treatment, Family Caretaker Enhancement, Case Management, Neighborhood Helping, Volunteer Linking, Mutual Help/Self Help, and Community Empowerment. The clinical treatment approach involves direct clinical intervention with the elderly individual as the client in order to assess and strengthen the support systems of at-risk individuals. The clinician assesses problems through a social system, rather than intrapsychic viewpoint and his/her role is not that of a traditional therapist, but rather one of facilitator and catalyst. Family Caretaker Enhancement involves intervening with family caretakers of the elderly to enhance family supports and to avoid undue family or parent burden. Case Management is a treatment approach in which professionals have major involvement. Its aim is to help address the issues of fragmentation, lack of accessibility, and lack of accountability in the delivery of services to older adults. Neighborhood Helping involves strengthening the networks of elderly individuals through enhancing their ties with natural helpers and community gatekeepers. Natural helpers are ordinary individuals identified by others in the community as being good listeners and helpers. Advantages of help provided by natural helpers include easy accessibility, lack of stigma, no cost, mutuality of helping, and its basis in proximity, friendship, and/or durability over time (Froland, Pancoast, Chapman, & Kimboko, 1981; Sauer & Coward, 1985).

A partnership between professionals and natural helpers can be an innovative approach to service delivery. Professional social workers can provide natural helpers with information about new programs and services and can also reinforce the work of the natural helpers. Volunteer Linking involves the creation of ties, usually targeted directly to individuals in need. Assistance is provided through a helper who is trained, supervised, and organized by a formal agency. Volunteer linking demands significant and continued involvement from professionals, initially in the recruitment and training of volunteers, and then in ongoing efforts to sustain the created relationship. Mutual Aid/Self-Help can be formalized to meet mutual support and guidance needs; service-exchange assist individuals to meet their needs through a formalized exchange of services and the creation of artificial networks through funded grants such as the Elder Program of the University of Louisville Gerontology Center. Lastly, Community empowerment is aimed at increasing the capacity or the group's ability to utilize power and to gain equity for elderly individuals. This model creates linkages between community and professionals helping networks. Professionals act in an advisory capacity to community groups instead of strictly as service providers.

Although these interventions are suggested for social work, some caveats need to be pointed out. Informal support systems should not be seen as a rationale to cut needed professional services as has been the case where needed professional services are indeed being cut to reduce federal and state deficits, and families, friends, neighbors and other informal service providers are being asked to close the resulting gaps. There is a real danger that such actions could seriously overload and weaken informal support systems. There is also the danger of romanticizing informal support systems and failing to realize that such systems are not always positive and can sometimes do harm as well as good (Sauer & Coward, 1985), especially if unmonitored.

There are also a number of obstacles that may limit full utilization of social network interventions. Professionals may not be knowledgeable about the role and functions of informal support systems or may believe that only those with professional education and training should offer help to people in need. Informal helpers may in turn be intimidated by professionals and may be uncomfortable interacting with them or may feel that they are taking over. Professionals may not have the necessary skills for assessing and nurturing informal support systems. Depending on the intervention, specialized skills may be needed in counseling, therapy, consultation, group work, or leadership development and community organization (Sauer & Coward, 1985).

REFERENCES

Allen-Meares, P., and Burnam, S. (1995). The endangerment of African American men: An appeal for social work action. *Social Work, 40*(2), 268-274.

Antonucci, T. C., Ajrouch, K. J., and Janevic, M. (1999). Socioeconomic status, social support, age, and health. *Annual New York Academy of Science, 896*, 390-392.

Auslander, G. K. (1988). Social networks and the functional health status of the poor: A secondary analysis of data from the National Survey of Personal Health Practices and Consequences. *Journal of Community Health, 13*(4), 197-209.

Barusch, A. S. (1999). Religion, adversity and age: Religious experience of low-income elderly women. *Journal of Sociology and Social Welfare, 26*(1), 125-142.

Berg, G. E., Fonss, N., Reed, A. J., and VandeCreek, L. (1995). The impact of religious faith and practice on patients suffering from a major affective disorder: A cost analysis. *Journal of Pastoral Care, 49*(4), 359-363.

Bertera, E. M. (1997). Consumption and generation of social support scale: Its psychometric properties in low socioeconomic status elderly. *Journal of Clinical Geropsychology, 3*(2), 139-147.

Billingsley, A. (1992). *Climbing Jacob's ladder*. New York: Simon & Shuster.

Boyd-Franklin, N. (1989). *Black families in therapy*. New York: Guilford.

Campbell, V. A., Crews, J. E., Moriarty, D. G., Zack, M. M., and Blackman, D. K. (1999). Surveillance for sensory impairment, activity limitation, and health-related quality of life among older adults–United States, 1993-1997. *Mortality Weekly Report CDC Surveillance Summary, 48*(8), 131-156.

Carter, C. S. (2000). Religion, adversity and age: Religious experiences of low-income elderly women. *Journal of Social Work Education, 36*(1), 79-88.

Cox, H. G. (1993). *Later life: The realities of aging*. New Jersey: Prentice Hall.

Dagnam, D. L., and Ruddick et al. (1998). A longitudinal study of the quality of life of older people with intellectual disability after leaving hospital. *Journal of Intellectual Disabilities Research, 42*(Pt 2), 112-121.

Daley, A., Jennigs, J., Beckett, J., and Leashore, B. (1995). Effective coping strategies of African Americans. *Social Work*, *40*(2), 240-248.

Daly, M. P., and Berman, B. M. (1993). Rehabilitation of the elderly patient with arthritis. *Clinical Geriatric Medicine*, *9*(4), 783-801.

Darrow, S. L., Russell, M., Cooper, M. L., Mudar, P., and Frone, M. R. (1992). Sociodemographic correlates of alcohol consumption among African-American and white women. *Women's Health*, *18*(4), 35-51.

Delgado, M. (1996). Religion as a caregiving system for Puerto Rican elders with functional disabilities. *Journal of Gerontological Social Work*, *26*(3/4), 129-143.

Dijkers, M. P. (1999). Correlates of life satisfaction among persons with spinal cord injury. *Archives of Physical Medical Rehabilitation*, *80*(8), 867-876.

Forster, L., and Stoller, E. (1992). The impact of social support on mortality: A seven-year follow-up of older men and women. *Journal of Applied Gerontology*, *11*(2), 173-186.

Fox, S. A., Pitkin, K., Paul, C., Carson, S., and Duan, N. (1998). Breast cancer screening adherence: Does church attendance matter? *Health Education Behavior*, *25*(6), 742-758.

Fried, L. P., Bandeen-Roche, K., Kasper, J. D., and Guralnik, J. M. (1999). Association of comorbidity with disability in older women: The women's health and aging study. *Journal of Clinical Epidemiology*, *52*(1), 27-37.

Froland, C., Pancoast, D., Chapman, N., and Kimboko, P. (1981). *Helping networks and human services.* Beverly Hills, CA: Sage Publications.

Gottlieb, B. H. (1985). Social networks and social support: An overview of research, practice, and policy implications. *Health Education Quarterly*, *12*(1), 5-22.

Guy, R. F. (1982). Religion, physical disabilities, and life satisfaction in older age cohorts. *International Journal of Aging and Human Development*, *15*(3), 225-232.

Heath, G. W., and Fentem, P. H. (1997). Physical activity among persons with disabilities: A public health perspective. *Exercise Sport Science Review*, *25*, 195-234.

Heisel, M. A., and Faulkner, A. O. (1982). Religiosity in an older black population. *The Gerontologist*, *22*(4), 354-358.

Holmes, E., and Holmes, I. (1995). *Other cultures, elder years.* Thousand Oaks, CA: Sage Publications.

Idler, E. L., and Kasl, S. V. (1997). Religion among disabled and nondisabled persons II: Attendance at religious services as a predictor of the course of disability [see comments]. *Journal of Gerontological Behavior, Psychological Science and Social Science*, *52*(6), 306-316.

Joseph, M. V. (1988). Religion and social work practice. *Social Casework*, *69*(7), 443-452.

Koenig, H. G., Bearon, L. B., Hover, M., and Travis, J. L. D. (1991). Religious perspectives of doctors, nurses, patients, and families. *Journal of Pastoral Care*, *45*(3), 254-267.

Markides, K. S. (1983). Aging, religiosity, and adjustment: A longitudinal analysis. *Journal of Gerontology*, *38*(5), 621-625.

Ortega, S. T., Crutchfield, R.D., and Rusing, W. (1983). Race difference in elderly personal wellbeing, friendship, family and church. *Research on Aging*, *5*(1), 101-118.

Sauer, W., and Coward, R. (1985). *Social support networks and the care of the elderly.* NY: Springer Publishing Co.

Siebert, D., Mutran, E., and Reitzes, D. (1999). Friendship and social support: The importance of role identity to aging adults. *Journal of Social Work, 44*(6), 522-533.

Suarez, L., Lloyd, L., Weiss, N., Rainbolt, T., and Pulley, L. (1994). Effect of social networks on cancer-screening behavior of older Mexican-American women. *Journal of National Cancer Institute, 86*(10), 775-779.

U.S. Dept. Health and Human Services. (July 1997). *National Health and Nutrition Examination Survey, III 1988-94* (CD-ROM Series 11, No. 1A, ASCII Version). Washington, DC: National Center for Health Statistics.

Whitehouse, R., Shope, J. T., Sullivan, D. B., and Kulik, C. L. (1989). Children with juvenile rheumatoid arthritis at school. Functional problems, participation in physical education. The implementation of Public Law 94-142. *Clinical Pediatric (Phila), 28*(11), 509-514.

Young, G., and Dowling, W. (1987). Dimensions of religiosity in old age: Accounting for variation in types of participation. *Journal of Gerontology, 42*(4), 376-380.

A Logotherapeutic Approach
to the Quest for Meaningful Old Age

David Guttmann

SUMMARY. This article introduces logotherapy as a meaning centered psychotherapy and its relevance to social work with the aged. According to this theory, human beings are motivated first and foremost to finding meaning in life. Ways of discovering meaning are discussed along with Frankl's "tragic triad," consisting of guilt, suffering, and death. Each of these unavoidable factors in life offer opportunities for discovering meaning. The importance of spirituality in old age is stressed, and Cicero's Cato "the elder" is presented as a model for meaningful old age. *[Article copies available for a fee from The Haworth Document Delivery Service: 1-800-HAWORTH. E-mail address: <getinfo@haworthpressinc.com> Website: <http://www.HaworthPress.com> © 2001 by The Haworth Press, Inc. All rights reserved.]*

KEYWORDS. Aging, meaning, spirituality, logotherapy, social work

BACKGROUND

The dramatic growth of the aged population (65 years old and older) in the world has become a major area of study in many universities and

David Guttmann is Professor, Faculty of Welfare and Health Studies, University of Haifa, Mount Carmel, Haifa 31905, Israel.

Author note: This article is dedicated to the memory of my former Dean and much-respected friend and mentor, Professor Daniel Thursz, whose life is a model of meaningful living for all of us.

[Haworth co-indexing entry note]: "A Logotherapeutic Approach to the Quest for Meaningful Old Age." Guttmann, David. Co-published simultaneously in *Social Thought* (The Haworth Press, Inc.) Vol. 20, No. 3/4, 2001, pp. 117-128; and: *Issues in Global Aging* (ed: Frederick L. Ahearn, Jr.) The Haworth Press, Inc., 2001, pp. 117-128. Single or multiple copies of this article are available for a fee from The Haworth Document Delivery Service [1-800-HAWORTH, 9:00 a.m. - 5:00 p.m. (EST). E-mail address: getinfo@haworthpressinc.com].

research centers in the past two decades and continues to be a most frequently investigated subject in its complexity by many disciplines (Olsen, 1994). The sudden popularity of this previously rather neglected aspect of human growth and development is largely due to two factors, namely, demography and finances. As for the first, there is a new realization by social policy makers that the aged population of the world is growing by leaps and bounds. Already there are well above half a billion people 65 years old and older living on our planet (Thursz, 1998). In most industrialized countries the aged comprise from 10 to 15 percent of the total population (Olsen, 1994). The fastest growing segment among the aged are the 75+ years group. Their numbers and proportions will increase, according to demographers, well into the second half of the 21st century (Guttmann and Lowenstein, 1994), and will have a profound impact on existing services for them.

As for the second factor, namely the fiscal one, it is well known that care for the aged, and especially for the "old-old," those 80 years old and older, requires an ever increasing share in a nation's resources. For increase in longevity is not only a blessing, but also entails growing expenditures for the provision of a wide array of services, programs, and benefits for the aged population.

Despite the great diversity found among the aged, there are several elements pertaining to all of them. The aged as a group are among the poorest segment of society. Especially hard hit are the widows, the childless, the dislocated, and survivors of major calamities, such as floods, earthquakes, ethnic cleansing, and, for the Jews, survivors of the Holocaust (Cohen, Guttmann, and Lazar, 1998; Guttmann, 1994). These people require a large share of the communal resources for their care in their own homes or in various institutions.

The purpose of this article is to present logotherapy as a theory which has particular relevance to social work with the aged (Guttmann, 1996b). Frankl's "brainchild," logotherapy, is based on the idea that human beings are not helpless creatures tossed about by the forces of fate. They have the power, and the capacity, to shape their own destiny. In addition, their major motivation is to live a personally meaningful life–rather than to be left to the mercy of instinctual forces and to their unconscious urgings–as per much of the psychological literature indicates. Logotherapy's approach to the age old and universal human quest for meaningful life is equally applicable to the young and the old, to the sick and to the healthy, in short, to all of the population whom social workers serve.

The emphasis of this article is on the spiritual aspects of aging. These are central to people as they age. Logotherapy is one approach, albeit a major one, to spiritually meaningful living. Its major tenets complement social work's value base and attitude to life and to human dignity, as well as to its methods of treatment. Of particular importance for the practicing social worker serving the aged population is logotherapy's approach to the "tragic triad," which affects everybody, and which is more urgently felt in old age, namely, guilt, suffering, and death. Of these, much more will be said later. Logotherapy also offers ways in turning these factors in life into opportunities for discovering meaning. It is hoped that this article will motivate social workers to canvass the logotherapeutic literature and to become familiar with its major concepts and methods of intervention. These will no doubt enrich social workers' knowledge and professional practice both in a philosophical and in an applied sense.

AGING IN ANTIQUITY:
BIBLICAL AND PHILOSOPHICAL APPROACHES

The age-old wisdom found in Biblical and in other religious and philosophical literature in relation to aging is still fresh, still relevant, still valuable, and still applicable to both professionals and laymen. Biblical writers portrayed the aged in realistic and pragmatic terms. They were cognizant of the physical and the psychological changes that accompany aging. The obligation to care for the aged was anchored on the fear of the elderly from abandonment. The Psalmist's plea: "Cast me not aside in time of old age, forsake me not when my strength is spent" (Psalms 71: 9) echoes over the ages as a reminder that fears of abandonment are no new inventions of the modern age.

The Bible tells us after Sarah has died that "now Abraham was old, advanced in years" (Genesis 24:1). In addition, the question is raised, why does it say "now"? For Abraham was old even before the death of his beloved wife. The Midrash, or the rabbinical explanation of the Old Testament (Guttmann, 1996a), states that before Sarah's death, Abraham was already advanced in years, yet he was full of strength. But after Sarah died, "now he was suddenly old." As long as Sarah was alive she acted as a shield against his old age, but once she was gone there was no protection against the vicissitudes of life for him, and old age literally pounced upon Abraham.

In our times, many elderly people perceive their longevity more of a curse than a blessing, as ageism and prejudice against the aged have reached frightening proportions. In addition, less and less "Sarahs" are there to protect them. In the Bible, long life was seen as a reward for the fulfillment of the Commandments, i.e., the Fifth. Good physical and mental health for the aged is a Biblical imperative since life is treasured as sacred in Jewish religion and tradition.

CATO "THE ELDER" AS A MODEL OF MEANINGFUL OLD AGE

Meaningful old age in antiquity was described by the orator and philosopher Cicero (in Shuckburgh, 1969), whose wonderful little book titled "De Senectude," or "On Aging," can still serve today as a guide. Cicero had written it in 45 BC. He used "Cato, the Elder," an historical figure from ancient Rome, as the hero of his treatise. Cato became famous in Roman history by insisting: "Carthage must be destroyed" in every speech he delivered in the Roman Senate. Yet, for Cicero, he became the model of meaningful aging. For Cato was 84 years old when he died, an unusually long life in antiquity, and until his last day he kept his physical and mental strength and freshness and never thought of the approachment of death.

In Cicero's book, Cato tells his listeners that everybody wishes to attain old age, but when they do, they despise it for having "pounced" on them sooner than expected. According to Cato, there are four reasons why many people think about old age as a time of misery. First, that it prevents us from doing what we used to do. Second, that it weakens the body. Third, that it robs us of the pleasures we used to have, and fourth, that it is close to death. For each of these reasons Cato has an answer. He says: "Not by the power of the muscles, not by speed, nor by bodily dexterity are great things accomplished, but by wisdom, a steady character, and a correct judgment. In addition, in these qualities the old are superior to other age groups."

As for the popular belief about the weakening of memory in old age, Cato insists that if you don't exercise it properly, you may end up losing parts of it. Yet, he also adds that he had never heard of any old man who forgot where he hid his money! Old people remember what is meaningful to them personally. They can keep their mental powers if they don't lose interest in the world around them. And as for the loss of their physical powers, Cato says these are mainly due to their abuse in earlier times. Excesses of pleasures bring frailty in old age, destroy one's judgment, blind the eyes of the mind, and have no relationship to moral values.

Cato tells his listeners that successful old age can be attained by keeping a humble diet, by working in the field or garden, and by meetings with good friends. These do not diminish with the advance of years. No gray hair, and no wrinkles bring honor to the old, he claims, but living morally and doing good and decent things. Those negative qualities attributed to the old, such as stinginess, bitterness, and quarrelsomeness are shortcomings of character, not of old age.

As for the fear of impending death, Cato claims it is a pity to see an old man not discover in his long life that there is nothing to fear. For why should I be afraid? Either I will cease to suffer after death, or I will be happy. When the end comes, everything disappears. Only your good deeds remain. In addition, these deeds continue to live on with each new generation.

"TEN COMMANDMENTS" FOR MEANINGFUL LIFE IN OLD AGE

Cato's advice to the young of how to live a meaningful life in old age is just one approach among the philosophical ones. Another one is the "ten commandments" for elderly people everywhere, based on modern gerontological research (Olsen, 1994). These begin with the letter "S" and include the following:

- securing the economic means for a decent survival,
- safeguarding the physical and mental capacities,
- selecting the appropriate time for retirement,
- strengthening social ties to prevent loneliness,
- spending time in sports and physical activities,
- securing meaningful work options,
- sophisticating oneself with new technologies,
- satisfying scientific curiosity, to be up-to-date in one's profession,
- satisfying sexual needs, and obtaining warmth and joy,
- serving others, rather than withdrawing into a cocoon.

These "commandments" are expressions of the human quest for basic security in old age. They relate to some of the most obvious needs of people everywhere in this world. In addition, they are meaningful in relation to the historic, scientific and technological world in which they are living–willingly or not. Yet, they fail to relate to the most important need of the elderly, the need for a spiritually meaningful life. This need is seldom mentioned in the professional literature on aging, except in logotherapy, of which more will be said later.

AGING AND SPIRITUALITY

The needs of the elderly cited above are well known to professional services providers. But their more subtle, subjective, personal, emotional, and spiritual needs, which affect mental health, as well as services utilization, are seldom addressed by researchers and by policy makers. In addition, the innermost needs of the elderly are simply ignored. Chief among these is the need for a sense of security in this world, and reassurance that they will not be ridiculed, degraded, despised, and devalued as human beings by the younger generations when their mental capacities decline with the onset of senescence. Nor will they be abandoned, forsaken, and warehoused in old age homes.

Finding meaning in life in old age is closely tied to spirituality (Guttmann, 1996a). In its secular and religious sense spirituality lies beyond one's comprehension. It draws upon a person's inner resources, nourishes one's identity, helps one to come to terms with one's own aging, and to make peace with self and others. Spirituality communicates, contains and tames experience, and helps with all those things that we can no longer perform or achieve. Spirituality is a major element in "ego integrity," which, according to Erikson (1959), is expressed through the acceptance of one's one and only life cycle as something that had to be had and permitted no substitutions.

FRANKL'S LOGOTHERAPY AND THE HUMAN DIMENSION

One of the major roads to spirituality in old age is logotherapy, which stems from the Greek word Logos, or the human spirit. Logotherapy's shortest classification is that it is a meaning-centered psychotherapy based on a philosophy which focuses on human orientation to meaning. It is the brainchild, creation and lifelong contribution to science and to the philosophy of Viktor Frankl, acclaimed author of "Man's Search for Meaning" (1963). Frankl's logotherapy focuses on the unique and specific meaning of life which can be fulfilled only by the individual. What matters is the search for meaning, and not the by-product when one attains the goal of his or her search.

According to logotherapy, a human being is not a helpless creature tossed about the forces of fate. Rather, he/she is the creator of his or her own destiny. Frankl claims that life is not centered on gratification of the basic drives or instincts. Nor is it directed to the adjustment of self to the demands of the social environment. Instead of these, and sometimes in spite of these, human beings are motivated primarily to finding meaning in life. The theory developed by Frankl enables us to survive in this world even under the most trying of circumstances. Logotherapy teaches how to conduct ourselves so that we may be able to overcome pain, sorrow, frustrations, sickness, and even death. Thus it is a theory for the prevention of mental illness applicable to both the healthy and the distressed, to the rich and to the poor. Frankl (1963) stresses that life does not offer anyone pleasure or power, or status. Life offers meaning. And meaning comes from choices and commitments that transcend personal interests. It comes from reaching out beyond us toward causes to serve and people to love. People are capable of finding meaning in any situation (Guttmann, 1999). Even if we cannot change our circumstances, we can still change our attitude toward them. The "defiant power" of the human spirit, a term coined by Frankl (1963), rests on two pillars: on a person's capacity for self-transcendence and on self-detachment. Both of them are used in logotherapeutic treatment of psychogenic neuroses, especially in treating phobias and obsessive-compulsive disorders in behavior.

FINDING MEANING IN LIFE

The ability and the act of rising beyond and above oneself are defined by Frankl as self-transcendence. In the concentration camps, where Frankl had survived horrible conditions for two and a half years, self-transcendence meant embracing a self-chosen task, and an immediate goal, such as aiding a hobbling inmate over frozen terrain while on forced march to a worksite. Frankl (1963) states that any attempt to restore a man's inner strength in the camp was based first of all on showing him some future goal towards which the prisoner could direct his hopes for survival, something that only he could accomplish.

Self-detachment refers to the capacity to detach ourselves from outward situations, to take a stand toward them, or to find inner distance from them. It is maximized when it is carried out for the sake of someone or for some cause. As Frankl says, everything can be taken from a man but one thing, the last of the human freedoms: to choose one's attitude in any given set of circumstances. A human being can decide what he or she wishes to become. He/she can change and can control his/her destiny. This knowledge is critical for human survival. Human dignity can be retained even under the most adverse conditions. As the philosopher Nietsche has said: "He who has a why to live for–can bear with almost any how" (cited by Frankl, 1963).

When a person is unable to discover, recognize, and accept meaning, he/she finds himself/herself in an "existential vacuum." This vacuum cries out for fulfillment. If left unfulfilled, the person may pay a price in the form of a psychiatric symptom, such as anxiety, depression, apathy, or anomie. In addition, in their more severe form, these symptoms may develop into an "existential neurosis." There are many elderly people, as well as young ones, whose lives are meaningless: people who see no sense, and no real purpose to their lives. Even those who seemingly live affluent lives can become bored, restless, lacking a clear purpose, and ready to commit suicide because they find life meaningless. Frankl (1963) claims that we are not supposed to ask what is the meaning of life. Rather, we should ask ourselves what does life demand of us at every moment.

THE "TRAGIC TRIAD"–LOGOTHERAPY'S APPROACH TO GUILT, SUFFERING, AND DEATH

Pain, suffering, guilt, and death are no strangers to members of the helping professions (Guttmann, 1997). They are "used" to dealing with situations in which these ingredients of human existence manifest themselves. For in life, nobody can escape some measure of pain, some feeling of guilt, and, of course, no one lives forever. These Frankl has termed the "tragic triad" (Frankl, 1963). However, how we respond to this "tragic triad" is entirely upon us. Logotherapy is particularly suited to deal with issues of guilt, suffering, and death. For each of them contain many opportunities for discovering meaning in life.

The Notion of Guilt

In logotherapy there is an attempt to differentiate between three kinds of guilt: actual, neurotic, and existential (Sternig, 1984). Actual guilt refers to two kinds: "guilt by commission," resulting from some act that was committed and was basically wrong; and "guilt by omission." Many women in their middle years of life, for example, look forward to the joys of the "empty nest," to the freedom from their parenting functions, and the pursuit of individual goals and dreams–only to find themselves riddled with new responsibilities in parenting–for their own parents. In addition, many such caretakers resent the "fate" that forces them to postpone, or to give up completely, their dreams. They may experience strong feelings of guilt for their thoughts. Surprisingly, however, a review of the gerontological literature indicates a lack of studies that deal specifically with the subject of guilt (Guttmann, 1996b).

Neurotic guilt is felt by a person without committing any wrongdoing. What causes neurotic guilt is the intention, or the desire, to do something wrong. This intention has unconscious roots deep in a person's mind. For illustration: When someone wishes secretly the death of an aged and incapacitated parent, and the parent suddenly dies of natural causes, then the person wishing the death starts experiencing guilt for having "killed" the parent and may become obsessed with the sense of guilt. Such guilt has no actual cause, yet the guilty person cannot get rid of this feeling.

Existential guilt is different from both actual and neurotic guilt. According to Sternig (1984), it is a subliminal preoccupation–a sort of inner nagging, an inner experience of discomfort, of dissatisfaction demanding attention. When we act to fulfill this responsibility, we attain a sense of serenity and well-being. However, when we refuse to act on it, we experience existential guilt. Logotherapists deal with guilt by admitting it and by trying to change client behavior not only to make amends when it is possible, but also to learn from one's guilt so that the behaviors are not repeated. For guilt is looked on as an opportunity to change, to abandon old patterns of decision making, and to make better decisions in the future.

Logotherapeutical Attitude to Suffering

"Cancer can bite my body–but it can't bite my spirit" (Takashima, 1990, p. 51). Frankl claims that suffering would not have a meaning unless it was necessary. Thus, an illness which can be cured by surgery must not be shouldered by the patient as though it were his cross. For this would be masochism rather than heroism (Frankl, 1962, p. 113).

Suffering can arise from the meaninglessness of one's life, and not only from painful experience or an unchangeable fate. An empty life causes as much pain and suffering as the other two listed above. Frankl

(1967) calls this third type "a fundamental human suffering, which belongs to human life by the very nature and meaning of life" (p. 91). There is a purpose to this type of suffering, Frankl says, for it guards us from apathy. As long as we suffer, we remain psychically alive. In fact, we mature in suffering, grow because of it–it makes us richer and stronger.

Changing a person's attitude–from a preoccupation with his or her own misery to the opportunity to be of service to others, to those less fortunate–and redirecting the mental energy to discover new meaning in life is the logotherapeutic answer to suffering. The meaning of life is unconditional even in the case of intense suffering. One has only to discover the meaning of his/her suffering to bear it well. Without this discovery, suffering can turn into despair and self-destruction.

Attitude to Death

Spirituality takes on special significance for well being in old age, when one has to adjust to and to cope with the many losses old age brings in its wake. Simmons (1946), in his groundbreaking research on the universal interests of the aged, found two basic interests. In the many cultures he studied, the interest to extend life as long as possible, and the interest to withdraw from life when the time comes without too much suffering and pain, and with good prospects for an attractive hereafter stood out (Guttmann and Lowenstein, 1993). Frankl (1962) wrote: to those things which seem to take meaning away from human life belong not only suffering but dying as well, not only distress but also death.

CONCLUSION: TOWARD A MEANINGFUL LIFE

Meaning can be discovered in a variety of ways: by work, hobbies, and volunteer activities, or in what we contribute to the world. It can be gained by enjoying nature, arts, and the universe, that is, by a passive approach to life. Most importantly, meaning can be discovered through the attitudes we take toward our fellow human beings and toward God. The famous Lubliner Rabbi once said that God becomes attentive to the person who sings in the midst of personal troubles and accepts them good naturedly. Logotherapy can help people, young and old, to find meaning in their suffering, and to turn human tragedy to human triumph by changing one's attitude to what happens, or what has happened to them. The Italian writer Oriana Fallaci suffered from a "terminal illness" for some time, and was open about her bout with cancer. She insisted that there should not be a denial of the term "cancer" as the first step in dealing with this "creature" inside one's body. "It is not sickness, nor terminal illness," she said. "Rather, it is a living organism which invaded my body against my will. Now I have to wage a war against it. For either, like in a real war, it kills me, or I kill it. And people who have cancer should not waste away their time. Instead, they should understand that death is imminent, and they should cling to all those enjoyments that life can still contain. Even amid the greatest physical suffering, life retains its value. I would love to see a triumph of life" (*Friderikusz*, March 2, 1994).

There is a common bond which binds together all those who have suffered intensely, said Albert Schweitzer in his autobiographical book "Out of My Life and Thoughts" (Schweitzer, 1974). Yet, for each person suffering has a different meaning.

It is the caring for others–for their welfare, peace of mind, comfort, and consolation–that raises attitudinal values high above all others. This caring is what makes social work a helping profession in the fullest sense. In addition, making this caring meaningful for the old (and the young) is the aim of logotherapy.

REFERENCES

Cicero, M.T. (1969). (Also published as a Harvard Classic, 1909).

Cohen, B.Z., Guttmann, D. and Lazar, A. (1998). The willingness to seek help: A cross-national comparison. *Journal of Cross Cultural Research, 32*(2): November, 342-357.

Erikson, E.H. (1959). *Identity and the life cycle.* New York: Norton.

Frankl, V.E. (1962). *Man's search for meaning: An introduction to logotherapy, a revised and enlarged edition of From Death Camp to Existentialism* (preface by Gordon W. Allport). New York: A Touchstone Book.

Frankl, V.E. (1963). *Man's search for meaning: An introduction to logotherapy.* New York: Washington Square Press.

Frankl, V.E. (1967). *The doctor and the soul: From psychotherapy to logotherapy.* New York: Bantam Books.

Friderikusz. A Hungarian television program presented on March 2, 1994.

Guttmann, D. (1999). Logotherapeutic and "depth psychology" approaches to meaning and to psychotherapy. In G.T. Reker & K. Chamberlain (Eds.) *Existential meaning: Optimizing human development across the life span.* Thousand Oaks, CA: Sage Publications, Inc.

Guttmann, D. (1997). "Homo elector" and "homo paciens": Fate, choice, suffering and meaning in the works of Szondi and Frankl. *Journal des Viktor-Frankl-Instituts*, 5:1.

Guttmann, D. (1996a). The meaning of the moment and existential guilt. *Journal des Viktor-Frankl-Instituts*, 4:2:54-64.

Guttmann, D. (1996b). *Logotherapy for the helping professional, meaningful social work*. New York: Springer Publishing Co.

Guttmann, D. (1994). Meaningful aging: Establishing a club for survivors of the Holocaust in Hungary. *Journal des Viktor-Frankl-Instituts*, 2:1:67-73.

Guttmann, D. and Lowenstein, A. (1994). The graying of Israel. In L.K. Olson (Ed.), *The graying of the world*. New York: The Haworth Press, Inc.

Guttmann, D. and Lowenstein, A. (1993). Psychosocial problems and the needs of the elderly in mental health. In F.J. Turner (Ed.), *Mental health and the elderly*. New York: The Free Press.

Olson, L.K. (1994). *The graying of the world*. New York: The Haworth Press, Inc.

Schweitzer, A. (1974). *Ma vie et ma pensee*. Budapest: Kossuth. (Hungarian translation.)

Shuckburgh, E.S. (Ed.). (1969). *De senectude*. New York: St. Martin Press.

Simmons, L.W. (1946). Attitudes toward aging and the aged: Primitive societies. *Journal of Gerontology*, 1:72-95.

Sternig, P.J. (1984, spring-summer). Finding meaning through existential guilt. *International Forum for Logotherapy: Journal of Search for Meaning*, 7:46-49.

Takashima, H. (1990). *Humanistic psychosomatic medicine*. Tel Aviv: Dvir Publication. (In Hebrew).

Thursz, D. (1998). Paper presented at the International Conference on Jewish Welfare Services in Jerusalem, Israel.

Aging, Religion, and Spirituality: Advancing Meaning in Later Life

Gerson David

SUMMARY. We would not be relevant in the 21st century if we did not visit religion and spirituality in the field of aging. This essay first examines the agist society and challenges its present mind-set to dispel ageism and engage in intervention designed to enhance quality of living. It next moves to a consideration of *aging and meaning* and the role of religion and spirituality in advancing meaning in later life. It concludes with a brief discussion of meaning-making and soul-nourishment of the able-old and frail-old, affirming the value of spiritual development continuing throughout old age. *[Article copies available for a fee from The Haworth Document Delivery Service: 1-800-HAWORTH. E-mail address: <getinfo@haworthpressinc.com> Website: <http://www.HaworthPress.com> © 2001 by The Haworth Press, Inc. All rights reserved.]*

KEYWORDS. Frail elderly, religion, spirituality, aging, meaning-making, soul-nourishing

INTRODUCTION

We are living in a New Age–*an age of liberation, self-determination, and freedom.* Winds of change are blowing from all directions, disturbing every system, every organization and every human group. Some

---

Gerson David is Professor of Social Work, University of Houston, Graduate School of Social Work, Houston, TX 77204-4492.

[Haworth co-indexing entry note]: "Aging, Religion, and Spirituality: Advancing Meaning in Later Life." David, Gerson. Co-published simultaneously in *Social Thought* (The Haworth Press, Inc.) Vol. 20, No. 3/4, 2001, pp. 129-140; and: *Issues in Global Aging* (ed: Frederick L. Ahearn, Jr.) The Haworth Press, Inc., 2001, pp. 129-140. Single or multiple copies of this article are available for a fee from The Haworth Document Delivery Service [1-800-HAWORTH, 9:00 a.m. - 5:00 p.m. (EST). E-mail address: getinfo@haworthpressinc.com].

groups have been shaken and damaged by these changes. Some are resisting them. Some have been liberated by them. Yet, many other groups are struggling for freedom. The minorities of color are struggling against racism. The women are struggling against the domination of men and sexism. The old are struggling against ageism. All these struggles are linked in the global struggle for a new humanity. Together these groups have the potential of a new community-based social justice system of human compassion and selfhood. As liberated spirits, old people have a huge stake in this new community, helping to create it and extend it.

There are more old people living today than at any other time in history. They are better educated and healthier with more at stake in this society. Those over eighty-five are the fastest growing segment in the population. Because long life has become the rule rather than the exception and the collective meaning systems have failed to infuse aging with widely shared significance, we have become unsure about what it means *to grow old.* The late Maggie Kuhn, founder of Gray Panthers, better known as Maggie, led the group of older adults to refuse to accept "sociogenic aging"–an assigned role as nonpersons–whom society would relegate to warehouses and play pens.

This "roleless role," leading to a diminished sense of identity and personal worth for the older person, is the single most important reason to raise the issue of meaning in later life. We have been wrongly taught that old age is a condition of loss, a time to quit, a mandate to withdraw. It is essential to demonstrate that old age is not a defeat, but a victory; not a punishment, but a privilege. Old age is an especially important time to cultivate, elicit and sustain a sense of purpose.

This essay first examines the agist society and challenges its present mind-set to dispel ageism and engage in intervention designed to enhance quality living. It next moves to a consideration of *aging and meaning* and the role of religion and spirituality in advancing meaning in later life. As part of the discussion, the spiritual model of aging, offering differing views on aging highlighted by Leder (2000), are presented vis-à-vis the well accepted notion of good old age in our culture emphasized by Rowe and Kahn (1998) in their book, *Successful Aging.* It then concludes with a brief discussion of meaning-making and soul-nourishment of the able-old and frail-old.

DISPELLING AGEISM

An essential prerequisite for developing and maximizing options for a quality life that includes enhancing meaning in later life is to intervene in the most basic of all problems of old age. Ageism is a term coined and defined by Robert Butler as *a process of systematic stereotyping of and discrimination against people because they are old just as racism and sexism accomplish this for skin color and gender* (Butler, 1989). Maggie Kuhn astonished years ago that:

> We must shake off our old hang-ups and prejudice, heal ourselves of the brain damage that society has done to our heads, free ourselves and our society from social fictions about getting older and being old: (1) Old age is bad, a personal and social disaster; (2) Old age is a disease that nobody will admit to having; (3) Old age is disengagement from responsibility. It often begins with enforced retirement, a shock that some people never get over because they equate it with retirement from life; (4) Old age is mindless. Time for play and naps, when the mind stops functioning and regresses to senility, relieved only by bingo and soap operas; (5) Old age is sexless, with denial of our own sexuality. (Hessel, 1977)

As noted by Butler (1989), knowledge is the most basic intervention serving as an antidote to numerous erroneously but widely held beliefs. We need to counter the old dehumanizing images of old age with new ones that enable us to be comfortable with our bodies and continue to grow, learn and keep our minds and spirits vibrant as long as we live. Accurate information must be disseminated in order to discount the myths and stereotypes through which ageism is manifested in our society–agist birthday cards, agist advertising, jokes about aging, agist language, age discrimination in employment, etc. In the last analysis, people can become educated about ageism only when they get involved in projects that will raise their awareness and dispel ageism when they engage in interventions designed to enhance quality aging.

AGING AND MEANING OF LIFE

The study of aging and aging persons refers to the whole person who is aging and the aged. The wholeness embraces the physical, spiritual, mental, emotional and social dimensions of human growth and development. A segmental approach to the aging process will result in a restrictive, one-dimensional, ludicrous distortion of the older persons. The human experience of aging and growing older requires a hermeneutic approach whereby it may be interpreted and assigned meaning.

James Birren has been advising gerontologists to utilize the integrative role of metaphors with reference to spirituality in aging. Traditionally, the spiritual dimension of aging has been dealt with in disciplines such as philosophy, theology, literature and cultural history, the latter two from humanities. Inasmuch as a very significant part of gerontology deals with the study of human development and aging, these are important concerns for gerontologists, particularly in matters of issues such as wisdom and meaning. Birren rightly points out that the topic of meaning in later life involves socio-cultural and psychological discourse, as well as theological and philosophical discourse. These perspectives warrant integration with biological metaphors of aging, for example, in the area of health (Birren, 1991).

A holistic understanding of the whole person is a must for gerontological practitioners to improve the quality of life for the older person. Although aging is largely a positive experience for most persons, it is unpredictable and unique for each person. Many factors shape each person's health and quality of life. Human life with all its individual uniqueness and diversity continues to present opportunities for personal development and growth. The challenge for the older person is to engage fully the present and not to mourn the past and worry about the future. Each person's life history with distinctive events and experiences results in an older person who is remarkably and wonderfully individualized.

Aging can and does have positive features, but it also has negative ones. Many older persons, for example, have experienced losses such as health, income, role, status, competency, autonomy and significant others in their life. Yet, many others have documented positive growth of human character, sensibilities and spiritual maturation. As persons become aged, the one truly serious problem that emerges is to assess whether life is or is not worth living. An often posed question is: What is the meaning of life during old age?

Increasing evidence suggests that the crisis of aging and being old is a crisis of meaning (Moody and Cole, 1986). Enormous gains in longevity as a result of medical and technological progress have been accompanied " . . . by widespread spiritual malaise . . . and confusion over the meaning and purpose of life . . . particularly old age" (Cole, 1984, p. 329). An individual throughout his or her life is motivated to seek and find personal meaning in human existence. Older persons need a sense of meaning in order to continue to struggle and cope with the eroding and debilitating diminishments that aging and growing older eventually usher in.

AGING, RELIGION, AND SPIRITUALITY

The aging of the baby boom cohort, whose suspicion of authority was hammered out in their young adulthood, has been coterminous with the separation of spirituality from religion (Bellah et al., 1985; Roof, 1993). Increasing number of persons claim to be spiritual and reject institutional religion or organized church. However, if one examines what underlines spirituality, one finds numerous and varied definitions of terms.

A major disagreement concerns whether spirituality includes a transcendent object outside the self (Wulff, 1997), and if it does, whether that automatically puts it in the religious camp and its associated dogmas and history of destructive conflicts. Noting the great diversity of definitions of religion and spirituality among the public in general and scholars, Zinnbauer et al. (1997) undertook a study to examine how individuals in various demographic categories define religiousness and spirituality. Interestingly, they found no difference in the association of the sacred with religiousness and spirituality. Descriptions of spirituality most often included some reference to a higher power outside self. In other words, spirituality for many people retained an element of the divine. However, in casting off connections to religion, images of the divine risk becoming merely a mirror age of the self. That is exactly what Bellah and colleagues discovered in the 1980s; many persons who abandoned what they considered the narrow confines of institutionalized religion had individualized radically to elevate the self into a cosmic principle (Bellah et al., 1985, p. 236).

Zinnbauer and his colleagues, from their perspective regarding the separation of religion and spirituality, in which the former is *bad* and the latter *good* has resulted in an extremely limited view of religion. They urge scholars and researchers to study religion from a broader perspective, which includes spirituality as an essential element of religion (Zinnbauer et al., 1997, p. 563).

Victor Frankl's (1946/1984) vivid emphasis of spirituality as the human drive for meaning and purpose furnishes a psychological framework for understanding the intersecting dynamics of religion and spirituality revealed by the work of Zinnbauer et al. (1997). Frankl portrays spirituality as a motivational phenomenon often implied when people talk about being "moved" by their own spirit (and not in a Christian sense of the Holy Spirit). In a broader context, spirituality can be considered as a motivational-emotional phenomenon wherein people respond to the drive for meaning by seeking that meaning within the self, in a relationship with other people, the world at large, both secular and the sacred. Psychologically, emotion signals the presence of a drive and offers an evaluation of its fulfillment; thus we find people talking about spiritual experiences of connectedness as fundamentally emotional (McFadden, 1996).

Spirituality, while inspiring humans to seek the experience of meaningful connectedness, provides no language or belief structures for thinking about that experience or offering any guidance for its attainment. Further, spiritual experience, as comforting or overwhelming or subtle or magnificent as it might be, offers no way for people to come to terms with suffering as an intrinsic part of human life, nor does it articulate moral values that would underlie efforts to alleviate suffering whenever possible. Finally, spirituality, particularly in its present individualized form, does not bring together communities of hope and memory. Religion, on the other hand, provides language, symbols, ritual, beliefs, and a community to nourish human spirituality. Though religion sometimes creates stultifying structures that suffocate the spiritual drive for meaning, religion has traditionally offered human beings pathways to existential meaning as well as ultimate meaning. When energies diminish, active involvement with life becomes impossible, interpersonal relations are broken and socially valued productivity ends, religion affirms the continuing value of the human being.

THE SPIRITUAL MODEL OF AGING

Leder (2000) engages in a quarrel with "successful aging model" expounded by Rowe and Kahn (1998) in their book, *Successful Aging,* summarizing over a decade of MacArthur Foundation supported research on *What constitutes a good old age?* They conclude that a low risk of disease and disability, a high level of mental and physical functioning and a continuing active engagement with life are keys to aging well. Leder presents some differing views on aging including the ancient Hindu context of spiritual growth.

Leder (2000) appropriately points out *The Laws of Manu.* Mueller (1971) is one source of disagreement with the "successful aging" model. The Hindu text cited below penned around 100 BC to 100 AD presents a radically different vision, indeed an advocacy for *unsuccessful aging* from the Western point of view:

When a householder sees his skin wrinkled, and his hair white, and the sons of his sons, then he may resort to the forest. . . . Let him always be industrious in reciting the Veda. . . . In summer, let him expose himself to the heat of five fires, during the rainy seasons live under the open sky, and in winter be dressed in wet clothes, thus gradually increasing the rigour of his austerities . . . let him wander alone, without any compassion, in order to attain final liberation. (Mueller et al., 1971)

The *sine qua non* of the above Hindu depiction of the stage of old age is disengagement and the assumption of the renunciative role of a Hindu casting off the manifold roles and duties of midlife and concentrating on achieving union with God, the ultimate purpose of life. The spiritual model of successful aging, according to Oriental religions, began with the primacy of the transcendent, on the assumption that there is something greater than the "ego-self," be that called God, eternal soul, the Tao, Buddha-Nature, etc. Our negligence of thoughts toward afterlife is the result of our total absorption during the prime of our life on mundane things such as earning money, raising a family, and advancing our career.

Yet, with advancing age, we experience bodily decays, mental anguish, and interpersonal losses. Children move away, we lose touch with friends, and we suffer from the death of loved ones. At work, younger, more energetic and cheaper personnel are preferred. Thus age renders us all forest dwellers (in varying degrees, referred to in the Hindu scriptures above), deprived of our habitual identities, placed on the brink of an abyss or the transcendent.

While the Western model of successful aging assumes that the losses that occur during aging should be contended wherever possible to demonstrate the resolve to lead a healthy energetic life, the spiritual model encourages acceptance willingly of the "losses" of age as opportunities for liberation. From the latter perspective, growing old can be viewed as an advanced curriculum of the soul.

In *Spiritual Passages,* Leder (1997) discusses different traditions' routes to later-life spiritual wholeness. As already noted above, the Hindu renunciate launches a contemplative quest that is well worth honoring in our action-obsessed culture. Buddhists call our attention to the imperative need of facing and accepting death. The Jewish tradition, as exemplified in the story of Sarah and Abraham, speaks to later-life joyful and creative rebirths. Taoism reconnects aging to the cycles of nature. The Christian tradition focusing on Jesus Christ and Him crucified explores the loving connection to God and neighbors that can transform suffering into grace.

In contrast to the Hindu renunciate who sets off on a solitary quest, Leder (2000) gives an example presented by Native American Elder Audrey Shenandoah from the Onondaga Nation in upstate New York. The elder remains within the tribe taking on a guiding role. Through the gift of long life, the elder remembers, gathers, and preserves that which is of most value from the past. The elder has the perspective to be far-sighted about the future and to see the interconnectedness of all things. Thus, in traditional cultures the world over, the elder mentors the youth, provides direction for the tribe and presides over ritual observation (cited in Johnson, 1994, p. 194).

Leder correctly points out our need for older wisdom has never been greater. With increasing longevity, the number of older people is increasing rapidly. Instead of viewing the graying of America as a burden to society, we should view it as a resource to expand the pool of elder wisdom. For accomplishing this result, we need to support later-life spirituality. Leder (1997) designed a hypothetical "Elder Spirit Center" that could provide spirituality-oriented classes, retreats, resources and guidance for affiliates and visitors. This Center could serve as a live-in residential community for those who, like the forest dweller, wish to pursue spiritual development taking advantage of the "forest space" provided by the Center for contemplative retreat. Simultaneously, the Center, like the Native American example, allows one to remain in the community with others and serve fellow humans in the larger society. Also, it might offer opportunities for mentoring and outreach efforts designed to share intergenerationally the fruits of elder wisdom.

MEANING-MAKING, NOURISHING SOULS, AND OLDER ADULTS

Meaning-making refers to the process through which humans "select information, sort it, filter it, incorporate it according to whether it is interesting or pleasurable or dangerous and powerful to be approached or to be avoided" (Ashbrook, 1989, pp. 19-20). Soul-nourishing refers to that process that involves persons "finding the true self in an ever widening circle, first in the whole and then in God. This process is lifelong with the goal of 'solidarity with others' achieved as people become able to expand their world view and move toward inclusive wholeness" (Jones, 1985, pp. 186-188). Wholeness has to do with "setting one's heart" in ways that foster both commitment and connectedness as persons seek to know and live the truth in relation to themselves, others, creation, and One-Who-Transcends (Little, 1983).

As indicated earlier, soul-nourishing represents a way of emphasizing a lifelong process rather than an end to productivity (Vogel, 1991). The remainder of this essay focuses on how older adults develop, learn, think, feel, and act in ways that empower them to make sense of life and death and to grow in love of God, self, and neighbor. Because spiritual development often becomes steadfastly interconnected with issues of health and role changes in old age, attention will be given to the special circumstances of the able-old and the frail-old.

The Able-Old

Apropos, the able-old, the point of retirement and/or sudden widowhood becomes a time for dealing with disengagement from some of the most significant roles and the assumption of roles that offer challenges and opportunities to grow and contribute to the well-being of others and the world. John Bennett rightfully points out that older persons can and must contribute to personal, family, community and societal life so that "necessary disengagement need not become apathy or complacency" (Bennett, 1981, p. 145).

Maves believes that elders who *will* "inherit the life abundant" in their later years are called to simplify their lives, within the context of a consumerist society so that their lives can be liberating. Elders are called to accept who they are–as persons created and loved by God. Later-life is a time "to heal the bitter memories" and coming to terms with the "garbage of unresolved conflict, unfinished grief work and leftover anger." Additionally, elders are called to be "good stewards of our health . . . to reach out to others . . . to find a reason for being . . . and to see our life in the context of eternity" (Maves, 1986, pp. 137-141).

For Christians, helping persons understand and reaffirm their Baptismal vows as they move into old age means that this is no time to retreat from the world (see Becker, 1986). Their calling in old age is to continue to grow in faithful discipleship to the loving God. It can be a time to focus on "walking the walk" and "talking the talk" of faith in ways that make the world a better place. It is a time for exploring faith issues and questions; no question is off limits and living into the questions is more helpful than being given someone else's answers. It is a time to renew one's commitment to grow in one's understanding of what it means to love God, self, and neighbor.

The able-old are one of the greatest resources families and faith communities have. Here are persons rich in life experience that may be able to engage in meaningful ministry both in the life of the church and society on behalf of their community. One of the ways persons grow in faith is to *act their way into believing*. Opportunities to serve, taking serious account of each one's gifts and the needs of the faith community and world can be avenues toward faithful living. Persons who choose to find ways to care and share will discover as Sarah Patterson Boyle did that "a sense of belonging goes with putting one's ear to other people's hearts" (Boyle, 1983, p. 164). Older men and women can grow in faith in ways that empower them to become mentors and storytellers for those younger persons who journey with them through life and thereby bind the generations.

The Frail-Old

Frailty in later life can instigate struggle with the meaning of life and the purpose of suffering. The God whom Christians know in Jesus Christ and Him crucified answers human cries of *"why God? why me? why now? why this way? why God, why?"* with an assurance, that no matter what the suffering, God's love is ever present. To suggest that suffering is punishment by God and the failure to proclaim the good news of God's sustaining and caring presence in suffering hurts those who desperately need to hear the encouraging good news of the acceptance, compassion, and hope offered to all by the Creating, Redeeming and Sustaining God.

Religious hope is grounded in God's promise and the faith community to which one commits oneself. Carrigan rightly points out "The hoping person exists . . . within a wider reality that transcends him or herself. The lone person can only wish, for hope cannot be experienced alone, apart from the hoping community. The community is the sustainer and vehicle of hope, and human kind always hopes with, whereas isolation contributes to hopelessness" (Carrigan, 1976, p. 43). Frail elders have the potential to realize hope and ultimate meaning within the bonds of faith communities. These faith communities, however, must be ready to respond to elders' particular needs so as to enable them to continue to grow spiritually, notwithstanding the limitations of frailty. Spiritual wholeness is available to all persons, although the frail may need special attention to their needs by concerned persons of faith.

CONCLUSIONS

Today older persons represent a vast heterogeneous group of many different religions, racial, and ethnic backgrounds. They demonstrate varied approaches to spirituality in later life. The contention of this essay is that all persons, regardless of their individual difference, need to find ways of making their lives meaningful and of finding wholeness in their lives. Such development may occur in many different forms. The encouraging hopeful message is that spiritual development does continue throughout old age.

The time is here and now for the social work profession to enter into partnerships with other non-governmental organizations in the civic sector to initiate a much needed national dialogue concerning such issues as definitions of *spiritual services,* eligibility for such services, the availability and training of qualified personnel to provide such services and funding strategies within the larger context of delivering comprehensive services in the health care arena. It is incumbent on our part as human service professionals and members of different faith communities to make it possible for our older adults to grow in faith and spiritual well-being–that is, in love of self, neighbor, community and God–and make meaning and nourish their souls.

REFERENCES

Ashbrook, J. B. (1989). Making sense of soul and Sabbath: Brain process and the making of meaning. *The First Annual Levy G. Kearney Lectureship in Chaplaincy and Pastoral Care.* The Department of Spiritual Ministry, National Institute of Health.

Becker, A. H. (1986). *Ministry with older persons: A guide for clergy and congregation.* Minneapolis: Augsburg.

Bellah, R. N., Madsen, R., Sullivan, W. M., Swidler, A. & Tipton, S. H. (1985). *Habits of the heart: Individualism and commitment in American life.* Berkley: University of California Press.

Bennett, J. C. (1981). Ethical aspects of aging in America. In Clements, W. M. (Ed.), *Ministry with the aging.* San Francisco: Harper and Row.

Birren, J. E., & Deutchman, D. (1991). *Guiding autobiography groups for older adults: Exploring the fabric of life.* Baltimore: Johns Hopkins University Press.

Boyle, S. (1983). *The desert blooms: A personal adventure in growing old creatively.* Nashville: Abingdon.

Butler, R. N. (1989). Dispelling ageism: The cross-cutting intervention. *Annals, 50*(3), 138-147.

Carrigan, R. L. (1976). "Where has hope gone?": Towards an understanding of hope in pastoral care. *Pastoral Psychology, 25*(1), 43.

Cole, T. R. (1984). Aging, meaning, and well-being: Musings of a cultural historian. *International Journal of Aging and Human Development, 19*, 329-336.

Frankl, V. E. (1984). *Man's search for meaning* (Rev. Ed.). New York: Washington Square Press. (Original work published 1946).

Hessel, D. (Ed.). (1977). *Maggie Kuhn on aging: A dialogue.* Philadelphia: The Westminister Press.

Johnson, S. (1994). *The book of elders: The life stories and wisdom of great American Indians.* San Francisco: Harper and Sons.

Jones, A. W. (1985). *Soul making: The desert way of spirituality.* San Francisco: Harper and Row.

Kimble, M. (1995). Pastoral care. In M. Kimble & S. McFadden, J. Ellor & J. Seeber (Eds.), *Aging, spirituality, and religion.* Minneapolis: Fortress Press, 131-147.

Leder, D. (1997). *Spiritual passages: Embracing life's sacred journey.* New York: Tarcher/Putman.

Leder, D. (2000). Aging into the spirit: From traditional wisdom to innovative programs and communities. *Generations, 23*(4), 36-41.

Little, S. (1983). *To set one's heart: Belief and teaching in the church.* Atlanta: John Knox Press.

Maves, P. B. (1986). *Faith for older years: Making the most of life's second half.* Minneapolis: Augsburg.

McFadden, S. H. (1996). Religion, responsibility, and aging. In Birren, J. E., & K. W. Schaie (Eds.), *Handbook of the psychology of aging* (4th Ed.), (pp. 162-177). San Diego: Academic Press.

Moody, H. R. & Cole, T. R. (1986). *Aging and meaning: A bibliographic essay.* Durham, NC: Duke University Press.

Mueller, M. (Ed.). (1971). *The laws of Manu.* New York: AMS Press.

Roof, W. C. (1993). *A generation of seekers: The spiritual journeys of the baby boom generation.* San Francisco: Harper and Row.

Rowe, J. & Kahn, R. (1998). *Successful aging.* New York: Pantheon.

Vogel, L. (1984). *The religious education of older adults.* Birmingham: Religious Education Press.

Wulff, D. M. (1997). *Psychology of religion: Classic and contemporary.* New York: John Wiley and Sons.

Zinnbauer, G. T., Pargament, K. L., Cole, B., Rye, M. S., Butler, E. M., Belavich, T. G., Hipp, K. M., Scott, A. G. & Kadar, J. L. (1997). Religion and spirituality: Unfuzzing the fuzzy. *Journal of the Scientific Study of Religion, 36*, 549-564.

Examining Role Change:
A Qualitative Study of Catholic Sisters
Who Became Family Caregivers

JoAnn Meyer Burke

SUMMARY. Women in Catholic religious institutes are members of organizations that prohibited family caregiving until the late twentieth century. Forty-six women from 11 non-cloistered religious institutes participated in a qualitative study focused on understanding their parent care experiences from the perspective of role theory. Embedded in a society experiencing an era of extended longevity, the study participants appear to have expanded the role of Catholic sister to include the ministry of family elder care. *[Article copies available for a fee from The Haworth Document Delivery Service: 1-800-HAWORTH. E-mail address: <getinfo@haworthpressinc.com> Website: <http://www.HaworthPress.com> © 2001 by The Haworth Press, Inc. All rights reserved.]*

KEYWORDS. Role expansion, extended longevity, family caregiving, Catholic sisters

---

JoAnn Meyer Burke, PhD, LCSW, is Assistant Professor and Field Practicum Coordinator, Saint Mary's College, Department of Social Work and Anthropology, Notre Dame, IN 46556-5001.

[Haworth co-indexing entry note]: "Examining Role Change: A Qualitative Study of Catholic Sisters Who Became Family Caregivers." Burke, JoAnn Meyer. Co-published simultaneously in *Social Thought* (The Haworth Press, Inc.) Vol. 20, No. 3/4, 2001, pp. 141-157; and: *Issues in Global Aging* (ed: Frederick L. Ahearn, Jr.) The Haworth Press, Inc., 2001, pp. 141-157. Single or multiple copies of this article are available for a fee from The Haworth Document Delivery Service [1-800-HAWORTH, 9:00 a.m. - 5:00 p.m. (EST). E-mail address: getinfo@haworthpressinc.com].

INTRODUCTION

Women who are members of Catholic religious institutes and care for one of their own parents are deeply embedded in a major social issue facing North American society today. How will individuals and families as well as the larger systems in which they are situated adapt to the changing reality that more of us are living longer than ever before? Butler and Lewis (1982) illuminated this issue almost twenty years ago as he discussed an emerging longevity revolution. While our lives are now being reshaped as bonus decades are being added (Sheehy, 1995), social structures also need to adapt to this change as well (Riley, Kohn, & Foner, 1994).

As the population ages, increasing numbers of families are becoming involved in elder care. While family caregiving is a normative experience (Brody, 1990), the family caregivers in this study are unique. Not only were they not prepared to live in an era of extended longevity, most had little anticipatory role socialization for their family caregiving roles. They were members of Catholic women's religious institutes that had prohibited involvement in family responsibilities. Prior to the changes instituted by the Second Vatican Council in the 1960's, their dominant role as Catholic sisters had confined them primarily to the social institution of religion; therefore, role conflict was minimal.

The aim of this paper is to better understand the experiences of female parent caregivers whose dominant role is in flux and who had little anticipatory socialization in early adulthood for assuming parent care responsibilities in midlife. The study participants were members of Catholic women's religious institutes in the greater Philadelphia area who responded to a request for participants for this parent care study. Among specific questions guiding the study are these:

1. How did parent care begin in the lives of these women?
2. What adjustments did they need to make in family relationships, relationships with friends, and relationships in the religious community during their parent care experiences?
3. Who helped them with parent care?
4. How did their dominant role as members of a religious institute impact their parent care experience?
5. How have they experienced ministry and the tasks of parent care?

The concept of social role was chosen as the theoretical perspective guiding this study because it provides a dynamic base for investigating identity issues for individuals as well as issues related to social structures and processes. Particularly important for this study is the concept of dominant social role (role centrality). Some roles, such as sex identity, marital roles, parental roles, and Catholic sister are more central to identity than other roles. All persons have one or several "master statuses" used to organize self-identities and by which we are primarily known in society (Merton, 1957). These master statuses prevent role overload and role conflict because they order behavior in specific broad patterns with individual interpretation. For example, in pre-Vatican II Catholic culture, membership in a religious institute was a well-defined master status that required a commitment of one's entire life to this endeavor. Since the church reforms of the 1960's, the master status of a Catholic sister has undergone vast change. It is not even clear at this point if it is a master status due to massive changes within Catholicism.

Role change happened suddenly for Catholic sisters as the Catholic Church reforms of the 1960's (Ebaugh, 1993; Wittberg, 1994) led to deep structural changes throughout the Catholic Church. Ebaugh (1993) says Catholic sisters are in the midst of immense change as they leave a highly structured way of life. Wittberg (1994) thinks the structure of the religious institutes is probably changing from a totalistic social institution with clearly defined boundaries to a more flexible voluntary association. In their study of the future of religious institutes, Nygren and Ukeritis (1992) found that members of these institutes lacked role clarity as structural changes were occurring in these organizations.

Not only is there ambiguity regarding their dominant role, Catholic sisters have also assumed more complex roles. After the church reforms of the 1960's, they were no longer restricted to the social institution of religion. They have become involved in a broad range of social institutions including their families. They are immersed in the social environment affected by this era of extended longevity (Riley, Kahn, & Foner, 1994), recent changes in women's roles (Moen, Robison, & Fields, 1994), and changes in religious institutes brought about by the 1960's Catholic Church reforms (Ebaugh, 1993; Wittberg, 1994).

The impact of the 1960's church reforms brought about a demographic shift in the religious institutes. A great exodus of younger members occurred from the late 1960's through the 1970's, and new entrants came to a virtual halt (Wittberg, 1994). The median age of the members of non-cloistered women's religious institutes in the United States had risen to 68 by the end of the century (Anderson & Co., 1996). The religious institutes severely felt the impact of the era of extended longevity.

As the members who stayed in the institutes reconnected with their families in the late 1960's, filial loyalty (Boszormenyi-Nagy & Spark, 1973) surfaced quickly into the action of the members to care for their own elderly parents if they needed assistance. It became possible for them to be involved in both their religious institutes, which function as their primary group, and their families of origin. Thus, women in religious institutes began to carry responsibilities for increasing numbers of frail elders in their religious institutes as well as their families. A systemic framework can be used to view this complex situation.

The family caregiving literature shows a trend toward broadening and lengthening its focus since its inception about thirty-five years ago. Earlier the field focused on the concept of the primary caregiver and was concentrated mainly on the negative aspects of the caregiving process (Kramer, 1997). Now caregiving is seen as a process that is dynamic and unfolding in the lives of adult children who care for frail parents. Moreover, the focus has broadened beyond one caregiving individual to the informal caregiving support network. Within the family, there is now an emphasis on dynamics that include attention to division of caregiving responsibilities and patterns of interaction within the family (Hirshorn & Piering, 1998-1999; Keith, 1995; Piercy, 1998). Moreover, attention is also given to other systems interacting with family members.

The loyalty concept in the contextual therapy approach (Boszormenyi-Nagy & Krasner, 1986; Boszormenyi-Nagy & Sparks, 1973) provides a multigenerational perspective that is helpful in discussing connections and conflicts that an individual may have within and between different relational systems. Loyalty involves attachment to partners who are entitled to a bonding priority. Not resolving loyalty conflicts results in a condition of split loyalty. In a condition of split loyalty, roles are also in conflict. Not only have Catholic sisters needed to address issues of loyalty between their families and religious communities, they have also needed to deal with role ambiguity resulting from changes in their dominant role of Catholic sister. The changing dominant role is more complex. No longer confined, Catholic sisters interact with multiple social institutions.

Lopata (1994) argues that role complexity does not necessarily result in role strain. She focuses on the problem of lack of adaptation in social structures and suggests that structural adaptation could ease role strain between public and private roles. Workplaces could offer more flex time, benefits could be available to both full-time and part-time workers, and retirement credits do not have to be tied only to the public sphere. These issues surface poignantly for family caregivers who need to juggle work and family caregiving responsibilities as well as plan for their own retirement. When middle-aged Catholic sisters have left their full-time ministries to care for a frail parent, some have experienced problems finding employment after their parent has died. In addition, retirement credits are lost during the time the sister is not employed. Members of religious institutes are experiencing the same issues with this dilemma as others in society.

Finally, adults who assume the responsibilities of parent care have been socialized to carry this responsibility as part of the role as an adult child, but there appears to be unevenness in this preparation. In the literature, life course studies reveal varied trajectories of socialization for parent care (Moen, Robison, & Fields, 1994). This has become more apparent as family caregiving studies have become more diverse (Kaye & Applegate, 1990).

This paper reports the findings from a study of 46 Catholic sisters who are experiencing vast changes in their dominant role (Burke, 1998). Simultaneously, they have assumed responsibilities for the care of frail parents and have needed to manage their roles in their families and religious institutes in a way that does not leave them caught in a split loyalty position without a clearly defined identity. Moreover, they are embedded in primary groups that were not structured to accommodate responsibilities for large numbers of frail elders within the institutes as well as large numbers of family elders.

METHOD OF INQUIRY

Because the aim of this study is to understand the parent care experiences of the study participants, a method of inquiry was sought that captures an insider's view of the experience (Mishler, 1986). A qualitative approach was used because studies of this type lend themselves to rich descriptions of patterns of behaviors and interactional processes as well as meanings people attribute to their experiences (Rowles & Reinharz, 1988). In-depth interviewing was chosen as the method to gather data because its purpose is to understand the particular experiences of the participants (Seidman, 1991).

Forty-six women met the criteria for the study and participated in the two-hour interviews. These women were members of eleven religious institutes. All women's religious institutes in the greater Philadelphia area were contacted by letter and phone, and twelve institutes agreed to circulate the letter requesting participation in the study. All study participants were self-described caregivers for an elderly parent. When the appointment was made for the interview, the researcher screened the caregiving situation to ascertain that the parent required some assistance with activities of daily living or instrumental activities of daily living. All study participants provided assistance to a parent. Forty-one of these women were still actively caring for a parent at the time of their interviews, and five had been caregivers previous to their parents' deaths. The participants in this convenience sample ranged in age from 41 to 77, and their parents ranged in age from 76 to 100. Each caregiver was interviewed.

The researcher took time to establish the most trusting relationship possible with each participant. This was done in an attempt to enhance the validity of the study. Because the researcher could be getting socially desired responses, questions were asked in several ways. Moreover, the researcher circled back to questions later if there was any intuitive sense that the responses were not accurate. To address issues of reliability, the researcher needed to attend to herself as listener and interpreter of the data and had to be faithful to reporting the experiences related by the participants.

An interview guide was constructed that addressed four areas of these women's lives: (1) family member roles, (2) roles as members of religious institutes, (3) ministry roles, and (4) friendship roles. Each interview was tape-recorded and transcribed. The transcripts were coded, and the analysis was conducted by identifying common themes and variants within each of the four sections of the interview. After summarizing main themes and variants in each section, the findings and conclusions evolved from careful study of the themes and variations (Weiss, 1994).

One limitation in this study is the failure to hear from others in the care system. Parents, siblings, members of the religious institutes, and friends are noticeably absent even though they were part of the systemic framework. Another limitation involves sampling. Although a convenience sample was used, there were a sufficient number of participants and institutes represented in the study to offer a range of responses and provide validity for the findings.

FINDINGS

Encountering Parent Care

The study participants encountered family caregiving responsibilities in one of four ways: (1) sudden onset, (2) gradual onset, (3) through becoming a companion to a widowed parent, or (4) by being an only child. Each situation required long-term changes in their lives.

A sudden illness or injury of the frail parent or the death or disability of a parent who had been the caregiving spouse of the other parent usually precipitated sudden onset parent care responsibilities. This brought sudden changes in housing and ministries for these study participants as they needed to be near their frail parent until they could make a plan for care. Sr. Mary Francis, age 52, related that she was not prepared for parent care.

> My ministry is spiritual direction. . . . I went on retreat in August. . . . In retreat, you always ask the Lord what's on the agenda for the next go around. . . . I'm always discerning what I am supposed to be doing . . . in September I went home to visit my father. He had a doctor's appointment and I went with him . . . he had a mass in his lungs and the doctor said he had only about six months to live. . . . I felt like I was shot out of a cannon.

The women who entered parent care gradually had more time to plan changes in housing and ministries. Others gradually drifted into parent care and made these changes later. If possible, these women looked for ministry opportunities that offered job flexibility so they could be available to parents when needed. In addition, they had time to reflect on issues of co-residing in the parental home or living in a convent or apartment with other Catholic sisters and commuting for caregiving. If they were commuting caregivers, they often looked for living situations where their absence would not create problems. Sr. Julia offers an example of being involved in care of each parent. She gradually moved to her parents' home and has continued to retain her teaching ministry.

> My father was sick . . . first memory loss in the early 1970's, and I asked to be transferred closer to them then. . . . I had a full teaching schedule so I would come home on Saturday and stay overnight through Sunday. . . . He kept getting worse. . . . Then I started coming to help him get to bed and was staying there every night. . . . By 1987, I discerned with my provincial that it would be a good idea to live at home and keep my teaching job. . . . After he died, I stayed on with Mom because she has glaucoma and emphysema . . . so I continue to live with her and have kept my full-time teaching ministry . . .

A third group of caregivers appeared to drift gradually into parent care, but this happened differently from the gradual onset described above. These caregivers became companions to their widowed parents after the other parent had died. The parents were not functionally disabled when their daughters began to spend weekends at home with them. Over time, emotional dependencies grew, and these women found themselves in enmeshed relationships with widowed parents. Some of the women realized they were caught in these relationships and sought therapy. By the time some of the women realized they were in these enmeshed relationships, their parents had become functionally dependent. In contrast to the women who sought therapy to deal with enmeshment with parents, others never realized their situation and would have to face it after the death of the parent. Sr. Jackie shared her experience with her mother.

> I care for my mother who is 86 and now really needs assistance . . . the pressure for my presence got worse after my father died because my mother was very dependent and her life centered around me . . . vacation, traveling, visiting. . . . I'd do it differently if I were going through it again. I knew it was happening but I didn't know what to do about it. . . .

The fourth group of caregivers was only children. They appeared aware of their responsibilities for their parents at a much younger age than the other women in the study. At the time they assumed their dominant role as Catholic sister, they were quite aware of having no siblings to help care for parents. They seemed to place themselves in a unique category in their religious institutes. They had been aware when they entered that they might have to deal with family care issues. Nevertheless, this was not addressed directly. Sr. Donna, who entered her religious institute when she was 17, described her situation as an only child.

> I knew I was it. I knew my parents had nobody but me if they needed care. I always thought I would just leave and go home with my parents if they needed me. Then, I'd just hope that the community would take me back after my parents died. . . . Of course, we weren't allowed to go home, so I just never talked about what I would do if my parents needed me, but I always knew.

Furthermore, only children talked about a dreaded loss of family when parents die. Those with siblings have some family continuity because there are still family members with whom they can interact, and those siblings can keep parental possessions in the family. Sr. Andrea, an only child who is caring for her widowed mother, described these issues of loss.

> When my mother dies, it will be harder for me than my father's death because after he died, most things stayed the same for me. But when my mother dies, I'll have to sell that house and those roots. . . . I have to sell my roots, my mother's and grandmother's china and silverware. . . . I'm dreading that . . . the community (institute) stands to inherit whatever I get . . . having no sibs makes it hard . . . it is hard to close a family home.

Even though these women encountered parent care in different ways, all needed to find ways to cope with it after the need arose. While they encountered parent care differently, eventually all needed to work toward a long-term plan.

Implementing Parent Care

As the women looked for ways to care for parents, their attention moved to five areas: (1) negotiating division of care responsibilities with siblings, (2) incorporating friends into their parent care situations, (3) finding transportation for parent care, (4) deciding where to live, and (5) locating and using formal care resources.

The researcher first became aware of particular issues related to the division of care responsibilities with siblings while working with Catholic sisters and their families in family therapy (Carmichael & Burke, 1993). The sisters thought their families expected them to be more available for parent care responsibilities than their other siblings. This is consistent with the literature regarding unmarried women's involvement in parent care, because single women are seen as having less competing obligations than their married siblings (Allen, 1989; Brody, 1990). Furthermore, the study participants reported that their siblings thought it easier for them to leave their jobs to care for parents because their religious institutes would care for them whether they were employed or not.

This left the study participants in an ambiguous position with their siblings. In one way, their families considered them as single women with no responsibilities in their religious institutes. Yet, the families expected the religious institutes to provide for their needs so they could be available to care for parents. Therefore, issues regarding negotiations with families took the form of both inter-role and intra-role conflict. Management of inter-role conflict involved being clear about what resources the Catholic sister could bring to family caregiving. Intra-role conflict management dealt with the negotiation of resources siblings could bring to the care situation.

Sr. Miriam noticed that she had taken more family responsibility than her biological sister. Although she acknowledges this, she is not sure why it has happened. She struggled to negotiate parent care responsibilities with her family since her dominant role of Catholic sister no longer defined her involvement in the family. The sisters focusing on inter-role issues must resolve the lack of clarity regarding the role of Catholic sister. If this resolution does not happen, they may spend their time in parent care in a state of role ambiguity, experiencing the complexity of roles as conflict.

> I am caring for both of my parents. I have only a sister and she works and has a family. What I have noticed is that when there is a religious available, sometimes the feeling is that she is not in a real job and her hours are negotiable. My sister is wonderful but by far, I have taken the lead. . . . I really get worn sometimes. . . .

Friends were another significant aspect of the long-term plan of care. Some friends offered "hands-on" assistance in the caregiving responsibilities as well as emotional support. Others were mostly available for emotional support. With prolonged parent care, some of the women suffered isolation and perceived loss of friends. Sr. Mary Elizabeth related her experience.

> . . . before I did not understand why people who were in caregiving could not find time to be with their friends. . . . I watch the clock when I visit my friends, you have to overcome the fear of letting someone stay with your parent when you go out . . . it is still very difficult to stay in touch with friends except by phone.

Part of the implementation of parent care involved not only negotiation of responsibilities with family and friends but also negotiation of use of institute resources. Transportation for parent care was one of the most difficult issues for almost all women studied. Most of the caregivers who did not reside in the parental home lived in convents where cars were shared. They did not have enough access to these shared vehicles to meet their transportation needs. They could not take a convent car every weekend to go to the home of their parents for caregiving. Furthermore, when the cars were being used by other sisters, they had no transportation available if their parents had an emergency. Some of the commuting caregivers used their parents' cars if this was possible and kept them at the convents so they could go back and forth to their parents' homes. In a few instances, the religious institutes provided cars to co-residing caregivers. Lack of adequate transportation was almost a universal problem for these family caregivers. Structurally, most religious institutes have made no formal provision for transportation for family caregiving. Sr. Sharon described her struggle with having adequate transportation.

> I get to my mother's house by train . . . thank God the community pays for the transportation. . . . I take two different trains and then walk to my mother's. On Sunday, my sister's husband always takes me to the station . . . it is getting harder by train . . . sometimes I take things to her like cans of coffee and so forth . . . and it is heavy to carry those things.

Sr. Phyllis described needing to make sure there was always a car available at the convent.

> In this house we have nine nuns and four drivers . . . the older sisters have doctors' appointments . . . and we always need a car at the convent for emergencies that might arise. . . .

Another area of concern involved deciding where to live. Some of the caregivers lived full-time with their parents and were not employed outside the home. Others continued to be employed full-time or part-time. Those who were employed full-time usually spent weekends in their parents' homes attending to caregiving responsibilities. Even though most religious institutes mission to family caregiving only those who live with parents and are involved full-time in parent care, many commuting caregivers are quite involved in family caregiving and may be the invisible family caregivers in the religious institutes. Some of the commuting caregivers are involved in the daily care of a parent. Sr. Ve-

ronica appeared to be trying to find time to be with her local community
of Catholic sisters as well as being a teacher and a primary caregiver for
her father. She works full-time, lives at a convent, and commutes daily
to care for her father.

> He has needed more in the last year. On Saturday, I go over there
> and clean and shop. I help with his meals every night and then help
> him get upstairs to bed. Then I come back to the convent and sleep
> here each night . . . but it is a constant monitoring, wondering if my
> father needs me . . . sometimes I can do some things here in the
> convent like shopping on a Saturday . . . it is wanting to be in-
> volved in everything but in just little pieces. . . .

The other aspect that these women needed to address in order to
move forth with a long-term plan involved accessing health care and social services. This system was bewildering to most study participants.
Legal, financial, and tax matters were equally unfamiliar territory.
Moreover, some needed to deal with property maintenance and had little or no experience with this. Some had family members who helped
with these responsibilities, but others had to learn through frustrating
experiences. They had not acquired life management skills in legal, financial, and property management because their religious institutes had
handled these aspects of their lives. When the stress of inadequate
knowledge of such skills was combined with the need to find health care
and social services for their parents, many of the women felt overwhelmed. Sr. Andrea, an only child, described her frustration with financial and legal issues in parent care.

> My parents were both professionals and have good pensions . . . fi-
> nancial issues . . . tax shelters, investments, I don't have any prepa-
> ration for this. My mother does not have a vow of poverty, and I do
> . . . so I can't treat her like a nun. . . . I didn't know how to open the
> safety deposit box to get the cemetery deed out when my father
> died. . . . You know I'm well educated and middle-aged, you
> would think I'd know how to do these things, and it is humiliating
> not to know. . . . I need practical information.

Furthermore, these women had no direct access to resources of their
own to use in their family caregiving situations. As one sister said, "I
can offer only 'hands-on' care because I have nothing else to offer" because sisters have no assets in their own names and their income goes

directly to their institutes. Thus, these sisters could only purchase care and consultation for elder care if their families had the financial resources to do so. They seldom asked their institutes to provide concrete resources for their families.

Only one of the eleven religious institutes utilized the services of a long-term care case manager. The study participants in that institute found her services extremely beneficial. The sisters in the other institutes that did not have this service regarded it as a need because the case manager assisted with access to health and social services as well as financial, legal, and property maintenance issues. Sr. Jeanne, a member of the institute that had a case manager, expressed her appreciation for this resource by saying, "She sends us information every month on financial issues related to family elder care, services for home care, nursing home information, and if I needed more, I could call her." This professional case manager was available to work with sisters throughout the caregiving experience. She was able to help them discern their caregiving responsibilities with their families as well as assist them in finding appropriate health and social services to meet care needs.

Integrating Family Caregiving into an Accustomed Way of Life

Acceptance of family caregiving into the life of Catholic sisters has been an incremental process. Initially, most religious institutes required sisters to take a leave of absence for parent care. Slowly over the past thirty-five years, this policy has changed. When the policy for family caregiving is altered from taking a leave of absence to missioning sisters to family caregiving, family caregiving is officially legitimized for Catholic sisters. In so doing, the religious institute remains obligated to care sisters' needs. Not all religious institutes mission their members to family caregiving, but family caregiving was called a ministry by many of the women in the study. Although policies appear to be changing in ways that validate parent care as a ministry, there is a structural lag in the resources the institutes provide to support these caregivers. Seventy-five percent of the caregivers in this study do not think their institutes provide adequate resources for family caregiving.

Sr. Mary Eileen felt that the institutes needed to support the family caregiving ministries as they would any other ministries.

> With wisdom, we have to be open to know that the ministry of our sisters also includes the need to minister at home with families because God knows, they gave life to us. . . . It is not just up to broth-

ers and sisters who are married or single at home, that Jesus was the servant of all, and we should not place ourselves above our siblings by not helping with parent care. . . . A sister caregiver needs to be financially cared for as well as emotionally, physically, and spiritually cared for by her community.

DISCUSSION

The findings point to three major conclusions: (1) the dominant role of these Catholic sisters has expanded to include family caregiving, (2) these women lacked adequate preparation for the assumption of family caregiving responsibilities, and (3) they lacked adequate resources for family caregiving. Nevertheless, they became readily involved in the care of their parents.

The language of family caregiving ministry appears to legitimize the inclusion of family responsibilities into their role repertoire. Yet, the language of mission and ministry did more than this. It enlarged their changing dominant role of Catholic sister. While their married siblings keep their marital and filial roles separate, these women appear to try to maintain the dominant role of Catholic sister by bringing family caregiving into it as a ministry. Perhaps role expansion is a way to be loyal to both their religious institutes and their families. Initially the role expansion took the form of increased role complexity as they moved from their one-dimensional pre-Vatican II role into multiple role domains. While they needed to deal with inter-role conflict when they met role complexity, the conflict increases when responsibilities in their family role take the form of parent care. By considering parent care a ministry, their religious institutes remain responsible for their welfare, and it also gives the sisters a way to deal with severe inter-role conflict. Dominant role expansion ameliorates the stress of choosing family over religious life.

Moreover, the sisters enhance their life management skills repertoire during the family caregiving process. Several noted that they learned skills in financial management, handling legal affairs and property maintenance, as well as care of frail elders. These skills are brought back to the religious institutes and become resources for religious community life. The life management and elder care skills these caregiver ministers are learning may be valuable resources to the religious institutes in the near future if membership continues to diminish and the leadership pool continues to shrink. The complexity of their roles and their dominant role expansion may have unrecognized benefits for them as individuals and for their religious institutes.

The second conclusion concerns preparation for assuming family responsibilities. Basically, their dominant role as a Catholic sister precluded their role socialization for parent care. Most of the women in this study entered their institutes when they were in late adolescence. Even though there have been many changes in sisters' lives during the past thirty-five years, the institutes are still taking responsibility for most of the fiscal, legal, and property management aspects of their lives. Many women in the study were glad they learned some of these life-management skills in their family caregiving experiences, but intense role strain accompanied such learning. Structural adaptations in religious institutes that emphasize responsibility for life management skills should rectify this socialization issue.

Lack of adequate resourcing for family caregiving is the third major conclusion from the study. While some religious institutes are missioning women to family caregiving ministries if they are living in the family home and have no ministry outside the home, none in the study were missioning those who were involved in full-time ministries and were living in institute housing and commuting to care for parents. Yet these are the caregivers that may be experiencing the most stress. Remaining to be addressed are structural adaptations to bring an increase in instrumental support (health and social services) to community members involved in parent care. Access to professional geriatric care management services appears to be very helpful to those study participants who had this resource available in their religious institute. This resource provided by one religious institute assisted sisters in discernment issues related to family caregiving responsibilities as well as assistance in locating and utilizing formal health and social services. The long-term care system in this country is very fragmented and difficult to access. Religious institutes can support their sisters involved in family caregiving by providing access to professional social workers and health care personnel who can assist sisters in planning and implementing elder care with their families.

Lack of adequate transportation is a major stressor, and this was noted by every study participant. This is particularly a problem for the commuting caregivers who usually are not missioned to family caregiving because they have another ministry. The religious institutes have not been prepared to provide a car to each commuting family caregiver. These institutes have had serious issues related to caring for their own elderly members. Because they have very few members under age 50, care of their own frail elders in the institutes is a primary consideration. The administrators of the institutes seem to be overwhelmed with meeting the needs of so many elders in the institutes as well as in the families of their members. Perhaps there is a fear that it will cost too much to provide resources for these family caregivers and not leave enough financial resources for the care of the sisters. If so, that echoes some of the current social policy debates concerning meeting the needs of a growing segment of elders in this society. Meeting the needs of increasing numbers of elders is a challenge facing not only religious institutes; it is a challenge facing our society. Yet, an interconnected challenge involves identifying the resources inherent in an aging population by identifying more roles for elders in society.

In conclusion, parent care gradually became acceptable for Catholic sisters during the past thirty-five years. Two types of caregivers were found in this study. Co-residing caregivers are often missioned to family caregiving and live with a parent. Commuting caregivers usually retain a full-time ministry and live in institute housing while they care for a parent. Both types of caregivers appear to have expanded their dominant role of Catholic sister to include the ministry of family caregiving. This dominant role expansion ameliorates the tension between the family role domain and religious role domain. When family caregiving becomes a ministry, it is acceptable in the role repertoire of a Catholic sister. Yet, the religious institutes have not been prepared for the influx of needs to support these family caregiving ministries. Findings indicate that the sisters have a lack of adequate preparation and lack of adequate resources for parent care. Further studies could focus on the structural issues facing religious institutes as they deal with increasing numbers of elders in the institutes as well as increasing numbers of elders in the families of their members. While this study investigated only parent care, Catholic sisters are also assisting in the care of frail, elderly siblings, and this situation deserves attention. Moreover, family caregiving is not gender-specific, and study could also involve the family caregiving experiences of priests and brothers. The participants in this study surely demonstrate that this era of extended longevity is deeply impacting social roles.

REFERENCES

Allen, K.R. (1989). *Single women/family ties*. Newbury Park, CA: Sage Publications, Inc.

Anderson, Arthur & Co. (1996). *Retirement needs survey of United States religious*. (*Survey VI*). Washington, DC: National Religious Retirement Office.

Boszormenyi-Nagy, I. & Krasner, B.R. (1986). *Between give and take*. New York: Brunner/Mazel, Inc.

Boszormenyi-Nagy, I. & Sparks, G. (1973). *Invisible loyalties.* New York: Harper & Row.

Brody, E.M. (1990). *Women in the middle: Their parent care years.* New York: Springer.

Burke, J. (1998). Pathways into parent care: A qualitative study of Catholic sisters (nuns) who are caring for one of their own parents. (Doctoral dissertation, Bryn Mawr College, 1998). *Dissertation Abstracts International.* (University Microfilms No. 9907558).

Butler, R.L. & Lewis, M.I. (1982). *Aging and mental health* (3rd ed.). St. Louis: The C.V. Mosby Co.

Carmichael, M.T. & Burke, J.M. (1993). Caring for family elders. *Human Development, XIV*(4), 37-40.

Ebaugh, R. (1993). *Women in the vanishing cloister.* Brunswick, N.J.: Rutgers University Press.

Hirshorn, B.A. & Piering, P. (1998-99). Older people at risk: Issues and intergenerational responses. *Generations, XXII* (4), 49-53.

Kaye, L. W. & Applegate, J. S. (1990). *Men as caregivers to the elderly.* Lexington, MA.: Lexington Books.

Keith, C. (1995). Family caregiving systems: Models, resources, and values. *Journal of Marriage and the Family 57,* 179-189.

Kramer, B.J. (1997). Gain in the caregiving experience. Where are we? What next? *The Gerontologist, 37*(2), 218-232.

Lopata, H. Z. (1994). *Circles and settings: Roles changes of American women.* Albany, N.Y.: State University of New York Press.

Merton, R. K. (1957). *Social theory and social structure.* New York: The Free Press.

Mishler, E. G. (1986). *Research interviewing: Context and narrative.* Cambridge, Mass.: Harvard University Press.

Moen, P., Robison, J. & Fields, V. (1994). Women's work and caregiving roles: A life course approach. *Journal of Gerontology: Social Sciences, 49:* S176-S186.

Nygren, D. & Ukeritis, M. (1992). The future of religious orders in the United States: A Summary report. *Origins, 22*(15).

Piercy, K.W. (1998). Theorizing about family caregiving: The role of responsibility. *Journal of Marriage and the Family 60,* 109-118.

Riley, M.W., Kahn, R.L., & Foner, A. (1994). *Age and structural lag.* New York: John Wiley & Sons, Inc.

Rowles, G.D. & Reinharz, S. (1988). *Qualitative gerontology. Themes and challenges.* In G.D. Rowles & S. Reinharz (Eds.). New York: Springer Publishing Co., 3-33.

Seidman, I. E. (1991). *Interviewing as qualitative research.* New York: Teachers College Press.

Sheehy, G. (1995). *New passages.* New York: Ballantine Books.

Weiss, R.S. (1994). *Learning from strangers: The art and method of qualitative studies.* New York: The Free Press.

Wittberg, P. (1994). *The rise and decline of Catholic religious orders.* Albany, NY: The State University of New York Press.

Index

AARP (American Association of Retired Persons), 8-9,35-37
Able-old, 129,137-138
ADLs (Activities of Daily Living), 40-41,86,89-91
Ageism, meaning-making and, 130-131. *See also* Meaning-making
Aging and the aged
  caregiver responsibilities, 33-45. *See also* Caregiver responsibilities
  myths *vs.* realities of, 5-10
  physical dysfunction and social participation, 2,97-115. *See also* Physical dysfunction and social participation
  programs for, policy issues of. *See* Policy issues
  retirement patterns and, 2,25-32. *See also* Retirement patterns
  social and moral meanings of, 1-16. *See also* Social and moral meanings
  spiritual and religious considerations
    Catholic religious as family caregivers, 78,141-157. *See also* Catholic religious as family caregivers
    logotherapeutics, 78,117-128. *See also* Logotherapeutics
    meaning-making, 78,129-140. *See also* Meaning-making
    nursing home adjustment and, 2, 79-96. *See also* Nursing home adjustment

zakat system, Pakistan, 2,47-75, 77. *See also* Zakat system, Pakistan
Ahearn, F.L., xi-xii, 1-2,77-78
AIDS (Acquired Immunodeficiency Syndrome), 4

Bailey-Etta, B., 77-78,97-115
Belief systems. *See* Spiritual and religious considerations
Bertera, E.M., 77-78,97-115
Birren, J., 132
B'nai B'rith International, xii
Burke, J.M., 78,141-157
Butler, R., 130-131

Caregiver responsibilities
  Catholic religious as family caregivers, 78,141-157. *See also* Catholic religious as family caregivers
  dependent elderly, definition of, 35
  family roles of, 35-37
  formal services roles
    comparisons of, 41-44
    in Israel, 40-41
    in the United Kingdom, 38-40
    in the United States, 37-38
    introduction to, 2,33-34
    reference and research literature about, 44-45
Caregivers Recognition and Services Act, 39
Case Western University, 2,25
Catholic religious as family caregivers
  contextual therapy and, 144-145

demographics of, 145-146
implications of, 154-156
introduction to, 78,141-145
parent care experiences of
    implementation of care, 149-153
    initial encounters, 146-149
    integration, caregiving and reli-
        gious life, 153-156
    role complexity and, 144-145
pre-Vatican II *vs.* post-Vatican II
    roles, 154
reference and research literature
    about, 156-157
Catholic University of America, Interna-
    tional Center on Global Aging,
    xi-xii, 1-2,47,77-78, 97
Cato "the elder," 117-128
Census Bureau, United States, 15
Chen, Y-P., 2,17-23
Cicero, M.T., 117-128
Clark, G., 2, 47-75
Clinton, W.J., 12-14
CLTCI (Community Long Term Care
    Insurance Law), Israel, 40-41
Cohabitation, 22
Community empowerment, 112-113
Confucianism, 4
Congregate meals programs
    Older Americans Act, Title IIIC-1
        (Congregate Nutrition Ser-
        vices), 4
    Older Americans Act, Title IIIC-2
        (Home-Delivered Nutrition
        Services), 4
Contextual therapy, loyalty concept,
    144-145
Cox, C., 2
CZC (Central Zakat Council), Paki-
    stan, 55-63

David, G., 78, 129-140
Demographics
    auxiliary Social Security benefits
        and, 19-21

cohabitation, 22
family structures. *See also* Family
    structures, 18-23
introduction to, 17-18
minority populations, 21-22
physical dysfunction and social par-
    ticipation, 2,104-109
policy proposals for, 23
reference and research literature
    about, 23
Social Security system, impact on,
    2,17-23
women, 22
Dependent elderly, definition of, 35
Dysfunction, physical. *See* Physical
    dysfunction and social partic-
    ipation

Elderly. *See* Aging and the aged
European Union countries, retirement
    patterns and pension policies
    of, 2,25-32. *See also* Retire-
    ment patterns; Policy issues

Family Medical Leave Act, 38
Family structures
    auxiliary Social Security benefits
        and, 19-21,23
    cohabitation and, 22-23
    demographic changes, impact on,
        17-19
    introduction to, 2,17-18
    minority populations and, 21-22
    women and, 22
Federal Interagency Forum on Aging
    Related Statistics, 9
Frail-old, 129,138-139
Frankl, V., tragic triad concept, 78,
    117-128

Generation X, 4

Gerontological Society of America, 79
Guttman, D., 78,117-128

Haifa University, 78,117
HCFA, 37
Hokenstad, M.C., 2,25-32

Integration, caregiving and religious
  life, 153-156
International Federation on Aging, 1-2,4
International Year of the Older Person, 8
Islam, zakat system, 2,47-75,77. *See
  also* Zakat system, Pakistan
Israel, formal services for caregiver re-
  sponsibilities, 40-41

JASC (Jewish Communal Service As-
  sociation), xii
Jewish elderly
  Jewish Home and Hospital, Bronx,
    New York, 77,79
  nursing home adjustment, impact of
    religion and spirituality, 2,
    82-94. *See also* Nursing
    home adjustment
Johansson, L., 2,25-32

Logotherapeutics
  vs. Biblical approaches, 119-120
  human dimensions and, 122-123
  introduction to, 78,117-119
  meaning in life, search for, 78,
    123-124,126-127
  vs. philosophical approaches,
    119-120
  reference and research literature
    about, 127-128
  self-transcendence and, 123-124
  spirituality and, 122

ten commandments for meaningful
  life in old age, 121-122
tragic triad (guilt, suffering, and
  death) and
  death, 126
  guilt, 124-125
  introduction to, 124
  suffering, 125-126
Longevity, social and moral meanings
  of, 1-16. *See also* Social and
  moral meanings
Loyalty concept, contextual therapy,
  144-145
LZCs (Local Zakat Committees), Pakistan, 49-51

Meaning-making
  ageism and, 130-131
  aging and, 131-132
  future perspectives of, 139
  holistic approaches to, 132
  introduction to, 78,129-130
  logotherapeutic approach, 78,
    123-124,126-127. *See also*
    Logotherapeutics
  moral and social, 1-16. *See also* So-
    cial and moral meanings
  reference and research literature
    about, 139-140
  religion *vs.* spirituality, 133-134
  segmental approaches to, 131-132
  soul-nourishing and
    able-old, 129,137-138
    frail-old, 129,138-139
    introduction to, 136-137
  spiritual models, 134-136
Measurement instruments
  ADLs (Activities of Daily Living),
    40-41,86,89-91
  Long Term Care Survey, 37-38
  MMSE (Mini-Mental Status Exam),
    83-84,87-88,90-91

National Health Interview Survey,
37-38
National Long Term Care Surveys,
37-38
NHANES III (National Health and
Nutrition Examination Sur-
vey), 77-78,97-115
NHRQ (Nursing Home Resident
Questionnaire), 83-84,90-91
Media, use of, 99
Medicaid and Medicaid reform, 43-44
Medicare and Medicare reform, 11-15
Minority populations, demographic
changes of, 21-22
MMSE (Mini-Mental Status Exam),
83-84,87-88,90-91
Moral and social meanings. *See* Social
and moral meanings
Mutual aid and self-help, 112-113

NAC (National Alliance for
Caregiving), 35-37
National Association for Home Care,
37
National Family Caregiver Support
Program, 14
National Health Interview Survey,
37-38
National Health Services and Commu-
nity Care Act, 38-39
National Long Term Care Surveys,
37-38
Natural helper-professional partner-
ships, 112
NCOA (National Council on Aging),
xii, 1-2,7-8
Network interventions, types of,
111-113
NHANES III (National Health and Nu-
trition Examination Survey),
77-78, 97-115
NHRQ (Nursing Home Resident Ques-
tionnaire), 83-84,90-91
Nursing home adjustment

ADLs (Activities of Daily Living)
and, 40-41,86,89-91
introduction to, 2,77,79-81
reference and research literature
about, 94-96
religion and spirituality, impact of
African American and Jewish elderly, case studies of, 82-94
case studies of, 82-94
introduction to, 81-82
measures of, 84-85
religiosity-adjustment-satisfac-
tion relationships, 90-94

Older Americans Act
reauthorization of, 14
Title I, 11
Title IIIC-1 (Congregate Nutrition
Services), 4
Title IIIC-2 (Home-Delivered Nu-
trition Services), 4

Pakistan, zakat system, 2, 47-75, 77.
See also Zakat system, Pakistan
Parent care experiences. *See also* Caregiver responsibilities
implementation of care, 149-153
initial encounters, 146-149
integration, caregiving and religious
life, 153-156
role complexity and, 144-145
Pension policies
demographics and, 26-27. *See also*
Demographics
in European Union countries, 30-32
future considerations about, 32
introduction to, 2, 25-26
retirement, reshaping and transformation of, 2,28-29. *See also*
Retirement patterns
in the United States, 29-30

work and workplace changes and,
27
Personal Social Services Research
Unit, United Kingdom, 39-40
Physical dysfunction and social participation
community empowerment and,
112-113
demographic characteristics and,
104-109
introduction to, 2,97-100
mutual aid/self-help and, 112-113
network interventions, types of,
111-113
professional-natural helper partnerships, 112
reference and research literature
about, 113-115
social participation characteristics,
105-109
social work, implications for,
109-113
studies of
findings, 103-109
methodology, 102-103
Policy issues
for caregiver responsibilities, 33-45.
See also Caregiver responsibilities
demographics and, 23. *See also* Demographics
for pensions, 2, 25-32. *See also*
Pension policies
social and moral meanings and, 10-14
of the zakat system, Pakistan, 2,
47-75, 77. *See also* Zakat
system, Pakistan
Professional-natural helper partnerships, 112
Psychotherapy, meaning-centered, 78,
117. *See also*
Logotherapeutics
PZC (Provincial Zakat Council), Pakistan, 49-51

Queens College, xi-xii

Racial/ethnic groups
nursing home adjustment of, 2,
82-94. *See also* Nursing
home adjustment
physical dysfunction and social participation of, 2,97-115. *See
also* Physical dysfunction and
social participation
zakat system, Pakistan and, 2,
47-75,77. *See also* Zakat system, Pakistan
Reference and research literature
about caregiver responsibilities,
44-45
about Catholic religious as family
caregivers, 156-157
about demographic changes, 23
about logotherapeutics, 127-128
about meaning-making, 139-140
about nursing home adjustment,
94-96
about physical dysfunction and social participation, 113-115
about social and moral meanings,
15-16
about the Social Security system,
United States, 23
about the zakat system, Pakistan,
74-75
Religious considerations. *See* Spiritual
and religious considerations
Retirement patterns
demographic changes, 26-27
future considerations about, 32
introduction to, 2,25-26
pension policies and
demographics and, 26-27
in the European Union, 30-32
reshaping and transformation of,
28-29
in the United States, 29-30

work and workplace, changes of, 27
Role expansion, 78,141-157. *See also* Catholic religious as family caregivers

Sasson, S., 77,79-96
Self-help and mutual aid, 112-113
Self-transcendence, 123-124
Social and moral meanings
　future perspectives of, 14-15
　introduction to, 1-5
　myths *vs.* realities of, 5-10
　reference and research literature about, 15-16
　spiritual and religious considerations about, 9-10
Social participation and physical dysfunction. *See* Physical dysfunction and social participation
Social Security system, United States
　demographic changes and
　　auxiliary benefits and, 19-21
　　cohabitation, 22
　　family structures. *See also* Family structures, 18-23
　　introduction to, 2,17-18
　　minority populations, 21-22
　　policy issues and, 23
　　reference and research literature about, 23
　　women, 22
　reform of, 6,11-15
Social work issues, 2,109-113
Soul-nourishing
　able-old, 129,137-138
　frail-old, 129,138-139
　introduction to, 136-137
　meaning-making and. *See* Meaning-making
Spiritual and religious considerations

Catholic religious as family caregivers, 78,141-157. *See also* Catholic religious as family caregivers
introduction to, 9-10,77-78
logotherapeutics, 78,117-128. *See also* Logotherapeutics
meaning-making and, 78,129-140. *See also* Meaning-making
nursing home adjustment and, 2, 79-96. *See also* Nursing home adjustment
zakat system, Pakistan, 2,47-75,77. *See also* Zakat system, Pakistan
St. Mary's College, Department of Social Work and Anthropology, 78, 141
Swedish National Board of Health and Welfare, 2,25

Takamura, J.C., 1-16
Thursz, D., xi-xii, 1-2,78
Title IIIC-1 (Congregate Nutrition Services), 4
Title IIIC-2 (Home-Delivered Nutrition Services), 4
Tragic triad (guilt, suffering, and death). *See also* Logotherapeutics
　death, 124-125
　Frankl, V. and, 117-128
　guilt, 124-125
　introduction to, 78,124
　suffering, 125-126

United Kingdom, 38-40
United Nations, 7-8
United States
　Administration on Aging, 1-3,8-9
　Bipartisan Commission, 34

caregiver responsibilities, formal
   services for, 38-40
Census Bureau, 15
Clinton, W.J., Presidential adminis-
   tration of, 12-14
DHHS (Department of Health and
   Human Services), 1-3,102
Family Medical Leave Act, 38
Medicaid and Medicaid reform,
   43-44
Medicare and Medicare reform,
   11-15
National Family Caregiver Support
   Program, 14
Older Americans Act
   reauthorization of, 14
   Title I, 11
   Title IIIC-1 (Congregate Nutri-
     tion Services), 4
   Title IIIC-2 (Home-Delivered
     Nutrition Services), 4
Social Security and Social Security
   reform, 2,6,11-15
University of Haifa, 78,117
University of Houston, Graduate
   School of Social Work, 78,
   129
University of Massachusetts, 2,17-23

Vista (Volunteers in Service to America), xi-xii
von Bismark, O., 5

Women, demographic changes of, 22
Work and workplace changes, 27

Zakat system, Pakistan
   changes to, 59-62
   CZC (Central Zakat Council) of,
     55-63
   demographics and, 49-51
   description of, 54-59, 77
   establishment and implementation
     of, 53-64
   evaluation of, 64-73
   future perspectives of, 73-74
   goals of, 64-73
   historical perspectives of, 51-53
   introduction to, 2,47-49,77
   LZCs (Local Zakat Committees) of,
     49-51
   PZC (Provincial Zakat Council) of,
     49-51
   reference and research literature
     about, 74-75